All in a Day's Work
A Collection of Reader-Submitted Stories

Kerry Hamm

Disclaimer:

Names, locations, and portions of the
details included in this book have been altered
to protect the privacy of those involved.

By now, I am sure you are all too familiar with my *Real Stories from a Small-Town ER* series, which were collections of stories told to you from my time as a registration clerk in Ohio. If you are new here, don't fret! You don't have to worry about a 'certain order' for *any* of my books, including this one!

I have since moved on from the hospital scene for the time being, but that hasn't stopped readers from submitting stories of their own experiences from the medical field. Over time, I have received hundreds of stories-some funny, some sad, some downright scary or grotesque-and have worked with my readers to bring these stories to you in a follow up to my last *Real Stories* volume.

If I've learned anything from writing my series and compiling this book, it's that none of us are alone. No matter how many Negative Nancys want to scold us on how 'nothing in this business is funny' (oh, shut up…yes, it is or there wouldn't be an entire genre available for the stories) or how we should all realize that 'these frustrations are part of the job' and should never be discussed, we're all proof that we've seen some pretty serious messed up things out there, right? We have seen the good. We've seen the bad. We've seen the downright vile and disgusting. And then, we've seen the humor in these situations and we've been fortunate enough to share them with one another. There is a certain peace in knowing that as no matter how crazy we feel, we have formed solidarity amongst ourselves, knowing that for every bad day you've had, others have had them too. We have worked through the challenges of getting up and facing another drug seeker, another child abuse case, another young death, and another 'how the heck did that even happen?' moment together. You guys are not alone, and this book reaffirms that.

Several of the stories have been edited to bring you clear-cut and clean versions of tales submitted by loyal readers. I have done my very best to edit out hospital and town names, and in some cases my submitters wished to withhold their initials and other details from publication or requested that I edit stories for grammar/spelling. Some stories have been edited for length.

Though some of the stories in this collection are horrifying, I am glad none of us are alone in what we've witnessed or experienced.

<u>What's Your Return Policy?</u>

I'm a nurse at a peds clinic, and I saw the cutest thing. I just wanted to share it with you. I know it's not what you're used to, but I hope you get a kick out of it.

A mother brought her newborn in for his six-week-old immunizations and wellness exam. She was accompanied by her eldest child, a bright-eyed four-year-old. Seriously, if I didn't know any better, I would think this girl just won a pony or something because she was so genuinely happy to be in the doctor's office, and it's such a rare thing to see these days from children.

Anyway, I called the mother back to start the appointment. Her little girl tagged along with a huge grin on her face. She didn't say much, but she was highly observant, noting the numbers on the digital scale aloud for me and helping me calm the baby when he cried at the sensation of a cold stethoscope.

I left the room and the doctor went in. The exam didn't take too long, but when the doctor left the room he asked me to prepare a prescription for eardrops and answer any questions the mother may have.

When I went back in the room, the little girl sprang from the wooden bench along the wall and handed me her brother's rattle.

"Now," she said, "it's important that you give this to his new mommy. He cries *all* the time. This is how to make him shut up."

I chuckled a bit. "New mommy?"

She nodded excitedly and asked, "This is where we go to give him back, right?"

I didn't know whether to laugh or feel bad for the little girl when her mother broke the news that the baby *was* going back home. The little girl sobbed for a good five minutes. I guess she was so excited about our office because she thought we were going to make her an only child again.

--A.P-R.

Idaho

PD Sounding Off

Your stories are cute, let's just say that. I, however, have been on the force for eight years and think I've encountered most of your patients and then some.

During my first-ever shift, I was partnered with a veteran pushing to retire. She'd seen it all, so when this 350-pound naked drunk woman plopped on the hood of the patrol car, I was surprised, to say the least. My partner yelled out one of those "Oh hell no," things and took the drunk woman's actions (and the crater of a dent in the hood) personally. After trying to reason with the non-compliant subject, my partner tasered this woman. The subject didn't fall to the sidewalk at the apartment complex. Instead, she fell back on the hood of the car, pissing my partner off even more. The subject was dazed, but she still had a fight in her, so my partner yelled for my help to take her down.

Well, at the time, I was about 150-pounds, about six-foot-tall; I was a bean pole-looking thing, no real muscle to me yet. I ordered the subject to place her hands behind her back, but she resisted. Before I knew it, she charged at my partner, but I couldn't get my gun or taser removed from my utility belt because I was experiencing first-time jitters. Most of the residents from the apartment complex had gathered around to witness the events, and I have to admit that I was nervous.

I did the only thing I could think to do at the time, which was lunge at the subject in attempt to take her down before she reached my partner. The sheer excitement must have taken her down because I know it wasn't my weight. I know this because the subject *stood up* with my legs scraping against her ribcage area, and my arms were around her neck, attempting to place her in a chokehold. I didn't think any of this through, so when she tripped over the curb and fell backwards, guess who got crushed under a heavy naked criminal? Yeah, me, that's who. The subject then urinated, with my body under her, so I was essentially urinated on during this takedown.

At the time, I thought the worst part about all of that is bystanders took pictures and posted them online. For months following the incident, the guys in my department printed out those pictures and hung them up all around the locker room, left copies by the coffee pot, 'mistakenly' left a few out while we were graced with the mayor's presence…

…And they put some in my glove compartment, which would turn out to be the actual worst part of all of this.

I had no idea they'd stowed copies in my personal vehicle, so I took this gorgeous, out-of-my-league woman out on a date and had to stop for gas on the way to the movie (I know, bad planning on my part). Well, while I was inside paying for the fuel, my date snooped through my glove compartment and found the pictures.

"My mom called when you were inside," she said to me, once I got back in the car. "She's not feeling well, so I think I should go check in with her."

Disappointed, I drove my date all the way back to her mother's house and tried to smooth-talk a reschedule.

"The truth is," she told me, with a grimace, "is that I'm really not into the kinky stuff that you are."

I was totally confused.

"What are you talking about?"

She opened my glove compartment and pointed to the pictures. I had to sheepishly relive my first call to a woman wearing this sexy red mini-skirt and try to assure her that I really *was* a police officer (and try to convince her I was a competent one). I actually showed her my badge and then told her to call the station if she didn't believe me.

Two years later that woman became my wife and is now the mother of our two beautiful girls (they get their looks from their mom, thank goodness). She tells this story when we have station get-togethers to anyone who will listen and gets a kick out of it *every-single-time.*

I guess not all of our crazy stories have to stay bad memories, huh?

--A.J.R.

Detroit vicinity

<u>Tornado Damage</u>

I was working as a phlebotomist smack-dab in the center of what is known as 'Tornado Alley.' My hospital had 45 beds but was usually full. We didn't have many 'slow' days.

Where I lived, we were accustomed to nasty storms. They don't call it Tornado Alley for no reason. I was lucky enough not to lose my home in the storms I rode out throughout the 11 years I lived there, but some of my neighbors weren't so lucky. Schoolkids actively participated in tornado drills around there, as did the hospital staff. We had designated 'safe zones' in the corridors, bathrooms, and patient rooms closest to the center of the facility.

The tornado that ripped through our town was an E-5 and it hit the hospital during my shift. Thankfully, lab was one of the few locations the tornado didn't hit directly, but the storm destroyed the emergency generators and we were left in the dark to find our way out. Three coworkers and I tried to navigate through the darkness and I heard so much noise that I couldn't focus on just one— people were crying and screaming for help; you could hear the building falling around you; the rain was still pounding above us. The rest of the hospital was destroyed. Staff couldn't move all the patients to safe zones in time, but it didn't matter. The roof was torn from the building in many places, even in those safe zones. Seven people died in the hospital itself. More than 100 other people in the town died as direct result of the tornado.

The worst part was there was no place for the injured to seek medical attention. Surrounding counties sent out their own paramedics and emergency vehicles and additional aid, but my hospital was reduced to little more than rubble and broken equipment. Surviving patients were transferred to surrounding hospitals.

My ex-coworkers tell me the hospital has been rebuilt with extra safety-features, but I saw the destruction that day, and it changed how I approach my life. That situation scared me out of the town and out of Tornado Alley.

--K.P.

Then Oklahoma, now Washington

I saw a cop use a stun-gun on a homeless guy who was masturbating in the waiting room when I was there for chest pain.

--V.C.

Illinois

Staff from Outside a Traditional Hospital

Kerry, I got ya beat on every story you've told. I worked back at this [well-talked-about New York psychiatric facility] back in the '70s. I started in '73 and lasted a lot longer than some of the others that started around the same time I did; I didn't leave there until '77, when I took a job offer at a place over in Connecticut.

This place was a disaster. I look at pictures of it now, since most of the campus has been abandoned, but I can tell you it looked relatively the same as it does now. There were 'paintings' on the walls, some done with wax crayons or real paints, but I saw a few done in blood or feces. When I came in, I was told the patient-staff ratio was 'much better' than it had been previously, but that still scared me. I was scared sh**less, like a lot of the nurses were, and I wasn't even a nurse. I was hired as a janitor while I went to night school to get a better job to support my wife and baby-on-the-way. I was often called by staff members to help hold patients down because if you were around, it was basically your job and your responsibility to ensure those nurses and doctors didn't get hurt.

Most of the time, I tried to keep my head down and do my job, just get through the day. It was hard. Some of these people would be strapped in a chair all day, and when I'd come back the next day they'd still be there, stewing in their own filth. I asked a nurse about it one time and that was the last time. She damn-near bit my head off and threatened to get me fired, and I knew I couldn't find another job that paid what this one did, so I accepted her reason that there were too many patients assigned to one nurse, and I left it at that. But that was a real problem around there. Patient life suffered because there were too many patients for the staff hired. I've done some research since this place became so popular, and I think I saw at one time they had over 5,000 beds and patients but only 2,000 nurses and doctors. It wasn't that bad when I was there, so I can only imagine that walking in that place during those years was nothing short of hell.

I wasn't there when it happened, but there were rumors that a patient escaped one night and the entire little community was thrown a curfew from the local P.D. I heard the guy killed a family. I still don't know if this happened, but I can tell you while I worked there that security was tighter and stricter than any other department there. I only saw one guy in that department *not* take his nightstick to a patient. Most everyone turned their eyes when it happened because there was nothing to be done about it.

About two years in, I moved up from janitor to orderly. I was assigned to the VIP floor, which was called that by a few nurses because it meant 'violent incarcerated persons.' I was the only orderly on a floor of nearly 100 patients. Several of them were kept in confinement, but there was an open part of the wing where the patients didn't behave any better. I can't tell you how many times I was bitten or spit on, and Lord only knows how many beatings I took trying to get some of these people to take meds. But I found a solution: I noticed a few of the patients watched as I popped Necco Wafers before starting my rounds, so I started offering a wafer as a reward to patients who took their medications peacefully. Before too long, I'd say about 85-percent of the wing reacted non-violently to me coming around with my cart. It took going home with bruises daily to maybe one-to-two bad days out of the week. The A&P cashiers must've thought I was nuts for scooping those candies off the shelves, but they helped me do my job without getting killed while doing it.

--M.T.

Connecticut

You Never Know Who You Know

I worked in a nursing home as a PRN on hoot owls. It was usually quiet there. I had worked there about two years and had gotten close to many of the residents. I know several nurses who are against getting to know residents, but I still cannot grasp how you can offer good care if you, well, don't care about your patients.

Anyway, I remember this guy being hired and he seemed nice enough, but there was something 'off' about him. None of my coworkers believed me when I said there was something strange going on with him. He had pleasant conversations with residents and then I also found out he was only PRN at the nursing home and worked at the hospital where I was shadowing on a floor for terminally-ill patients. Nobody believed me there, either.

During the man's first few months at the nursing home, two of his patients passed. Both were 'foreseeable,' as sickening as that may sound, and nobody batted an eye—me included. But I noticed some of his patients at the hospital passed as well. Again, nobody thought too much of it because a lot of the patients were respirator-dependent or suffered from terminal diagnoses of cancer or other illnesses. The nurses I was shadowing lost patients as well, so it felt silly to blame the man for losing patients who'd been hanging on by a thin rope. I still found this man most odd, and when I saw him my stomach twisted in the painful knots.

To be honest, I was relieved when I found out he was fired from both places. The 'official' reasoning from my bosses was that the man was often unaccounted for, but a coworker told me she saw him sneaking medical supplies from a cart on another floor and he was fired—at least that's the reasoning I heard around the hospital.

A few years later, I was watching TV with my daughter and we were flipping through the channels. Imagine my surprise when I saw that man's picture on the news! He had been arrested for administering lethal dosages of medicines to patients and was put away for murder.

I guess the moral of the story is not all the crazy stories come from dealing with patients. I've gone on to get my NP license, but I will never forget working with that killer.

--L.R.

New Jersey

Fashion Emergency

A mom brought her young son in during the middle of a rush on a weekend because he was stuck in a hairy situation and she didn't know what to do.

The young boy was forced into playing 'dress up' with his three sisters. They tried to put a dress on him, but his head became stuck in the neck-hole. When I stepped in the room, I suppose I first noticed how this little boy's nose was squished against his face that was being compressed by neon-pink fabric.

Admittedly, I laughed. This sent the child's mother in a fit of rage and she cursed at me much like you have described from your own experiences. I apologized and she did too. She said she was embarrassed that this incident occurred, especially since the two encountered their church pastor leaving out the same hospital door as they were entering. She didn't know how she was going to explain the incident to her congregation or her husband.

We were initially going to carefully cut the fabric from around the child's head, but his mother insisted we find an alternative solution because the dress was a pageant dress for his sister's upcoming entry. The boy's mother said the dress cost the family more than the ER visit would.

After asking a tech to join me in the room, we came up with a rather simple solution to the problem at hand. There was, in fact, a small button at the back of the neckline, that was still fastened. In all the frustration and panic, the child's mother had not noticed the button, and neither had I until closer examination. Once we undid the button, the boy was free to go.

--A.T.

Alabama

<u>Scary Submissions</u>

These stories were submitted by separate persons on separate dates, and as far as I'm aware, the persons submitting the stories were in no way related or in contact with each other. Once you read through a few, you'll see why the hair on the back of my neck raised after receiving the third submission.

First Submission, received late-2015:

I have been an RN for 19 years and feel like I've seen everything, for good or bad. The saddest thing I have ever witnessed was a woman brought in for abdominal trauma. She was eight-months-pregnant and was attacked. Her assailant attempted to cut the baby from the womb. I don't know how, but the woman lived. Her child did not. I don't know if her attacker was caught. I requested counseling for the incident and still have nightmares about that night.

On the opposite end of the spectrum, the happiest moment of my career also involved a child. I was not at the hospital, but was at a busy city pool. A three-year-old wandered away from his mother and she didn't notice until it was too late. Once she did notice, she panicked and everyone looked around, and only then did someone notice the boy had fallen in a crowded five-foot-deep section. Nobody knows how this went unnoticed, but when the lifeguards pulled the boy from the waters, he was blue. I was able to perform CPR and continue chest compressions until the medics arrived. The child lived. His mother invited me to his middle school graduation last month.

Something happened a few years ago that I still can't explain. It scared me so much that I transferred from the ER to Pediatrics.

During one 7PM-7AM shift, things were getting out of control. We received three ODs within ten minutes of one another, were already trying to keep a teen alive following a drunk driving incident (he was the victim, not the drunk driver), and we were short two RNs.

I went to the supply closet to get more tubing and was on the way back to a room when I passed the teenager's room, stopped as soon as it clicked in my head that something was not right, and slowly walked back to take a second look.

Standing on the patient's right side was a tall, black shadowy figure. To me, it kind of resembled the shape of a human being, or at least roughly. I could not make out facial features or body parts, but if you imagine seeing a person dressed in all-black, with black skin, black eyes—black everything— this is what I saw standing next to this teenager's bed. A sense of total fear engulfed me. This shadow stood there and appeared to be looking down at this young man's face.

I tried to call for help, but I was too scared and couldn't manage to make even the tiniest peep if my life depended on it.

Someone called my name and I looked away for half of a second. When I looked back to the room, the shadow was gone. I quickly told myself I was tired and had imagined the shadow-person.

By the time I had made it three steps in the direction I had originally intended to go, the alarms went off in the patient's room. I froze.

The patient's death was called a few minutes later. I'm now convinced that I whatever or whomever I saw was there to take that patient's life. I never told anyone what I saw because I thought they'd think I was crazy or that it would jeopardize my career.

--M.T.

California

Second Submission, received January 2016:

Local LEOs (Law Enforcement Officers) brought in a homeless drunk one night for disorderly conduct and disturbing the peace. His options were 'go to jail or go to the hospital.' I've been an ER tech for ten years and nobody's ever chosen jail, just so you know.

The patient was hysterical when they brought him to us. He kept yelling that the devil was trying to take him away, and he was fighting everyone because he said he needed to be discharged because none of us could save him. It was clear the man was dealing with more than alcohol intoxication. We paged our mental health unit for a psych consult.

The counselor couldn't get any information from the man besides what he'd been screaming, and after he hit her in the face, she and the ER doctors agreed it was time to give the man sedation medications. His RN drew up 5mg of Midazolam to start. That didn't do much, so he was also hit with a strong dose of Diazepam.

There was no doubt the dosages the patient received were enough to cause him to fall asleep, but he was still fighting tooth and nail—or as much as he could. By the time both drugs kicked in, he was mostly able to turn his head from side to side slowly and mutter that he needed to leave because the devil was trying to take him away. We made our jokes. We said how sad it was to see another patient in that condition.

Things calmed down and we left the patient restrained and sedated in hopes he'd sleep off the alcohol and then be willing to talk to our mental health counselor. We didn't pay too much attention to the patient, other than checking on him every hour or so.

I think it was about three or four hours after he was brought in that he sat up in bed, still cuffed to the rails, and screamed, "The devil is here," before passing out. Charge sent me in to check on the man, and I groaned.

As I was entering the room, I stopped in mid-step and lost my breath. There was a tall, dark shadow leaning over the patient. The energy coming from the room was frightening. Never in my life had I ever felt so afraid. The patient's pulse ox dropped to a critical rate and I was pushed out of the way by the crash cart team, who'd turned on the lights. The shadow wasn't there anymore.

The patient died.

I asked around later on that night to see if anyone else had seen anything unusual, but they said they hadn't.

I wasn't religious before witnessing this, but I'm happy to say I found a church and was saved. I really think I saw the devil taking the patient, just like the patient said was going to happen.

--P.A.

Montana

Third Submission, received early-2016:

I work as a CNA at an SNF (Skilled Nursing Facility) and saw the scariest thing a few months ago.

A Dementia patient started refusing to go to sleep at night. We administered sleeping pills but discovered she had been pocketing her pills (hiding them in her gum line to make it seem as if she had swallowed them) so she could stay up all night.

She didn't cause any trouble at night, for the most part. And she slept during the day, so we didn't try to force the issue of her taking sleeping pills anymore.

But then the patient started refusing to sleep during the day. We knew she was tired after the first night and day of being awake, but she absolutely refused to sleep. This woman was as stubborn as a mule, I tell you.

The head nurse rejected our suggestions to inject sleeping medication. Our boss said the woman would eventually fall asleep on her own and it was for the best that we didn't cause additional distress. She still wasn't being too much of a nuisance; she just wouldn't sleep.

It was day two of no sleep that this patient started trying to get out of bed unassisted. She made it to the hall twice and both times she put up quite the fit, telling everyone around her that she couldn't go back to her room because death was waiting. She was adamant that death had come for her and if she fell asleep it would get her. We tried to be nice about it the first time, just by speaking calmly to the patient and assuring her there was nothing in her room that would hurt her. The second time, I was assigned to sit by her and hopefully tire her out by talking to her about everything and anything.

The patient asked me to read to her from the Psalms, so I did. When I noticed she had stopped commenting on the passages, I looked up to see a dark figure directly in front of me, almost as if it were leaning over the patient's bed. I jumped out of my seat like it was on fire and screamed for help, but when my coworkers arrived, there was nothing in the room. Nobody believed me, either, when I told them. They all said I let the woman's 'hysteria' get to me.

The patient died while I was reading to her.

That was the day I saw death.

--K.B.
Michigan

Fourth Submission, received mid-2016:

Medics brought in an elderly man from a local nursing home suffering from visual hallucinations. This isn't as uncommon or out of the ordinary as a lot of people seem to think it is. We see this a lot in elderly patients with undiagnosed UTIs. Usually, once that is treated and the patient's medications are recalibrated, the patient is fine and is cleared to go back to the nursing home.

I was assigned to this patient and can tell you he was deathly afraid. Other than being scared half to death, he was completely lucid and polite. He kept looking up in fear and I looked up a few times to see, of course, nothing but the ceiling lights and tiles.

Finally, I asked the man, "What do you see?"

He said, "A black cloud."

I tried not to laugh, but a little chuckle slipped out. I couldn't comprehend how a 'black cloud' could terrify a person. I guess I was in a Disney-state-of-mind and was thinking he was seeing something cartoonish.

Anyway, I left the room to find the tech and get some assistance in adjusting him in bed, and when I came back with help, he was crying.

When I asked why he was crying, he blubbered something about the black cloud and was shaking so badly I asked the tech to inform the doctor of the patient's condition and ask him to assess the behavior so we could administer medication.

I attempted to assure the man he was in good care, but he continued sobbing and said he didn't want to die yet.

As I went to soothe him by stroking his hair back, the patient crossed his forearms over his face as if I was going to hit him and screamed, "Don't let it get me!"

I reflexively looked up and saw just what the patient had described: a black 'cloud.'

Seeing this caused me to call out a series of swears and I fell when I tripped over my own feet. When I told my coworkers what I had seen, two other people said they saw the same thing.

I did some 'research' about this and think it was some kind of end-life energy. The patient didn't die that night, but he did die a few days later. Rumor has it that a nurse on Med/Surg saw the same black 'cloud' looming over the patient's body.

--S.P.

Illinois

Feeling Hot, Hot, Hot

This isn't so much a story about the hospital as much as it is about something stupid that my own mother did to me way-back-when.

At risk of exposing my age, let me just say times were different then, and we didn't have all the fancy gadgets that we have lying around today. My mother was an avid Avon-customer and must have purchased just about every product under the sun from the door-to-door saleswoman, which must have driven my father mad. That's a little beside the point, but in our family of five daughters and no sons, our household could have produced a monthly issue of *Vogue*.

I was still a few years away from my teen years, but I still wanted to be like my three older sisters. They had the long, flowy hair, so naturally I had to grow mine out, too. They painted their eyelids and lips with mom's discarded Avon, so when I could sneak under dad's radar, I did the same. When my sisters lined up in the kitchen for mom to iron their hair, who else was in line but the second-to-youngest sister?

If you don't know anything about ironing hair, I'm going to tell you something about it. Now, we have these magical handheld devices that look like flat clamps and your hair is ironed on both sides at the same time. We didn't have anything like that growing up, unless you counted trying to achieve the same result using a curling iron. My sisters never used me as a guinea pig for that because if they were going to take an hour-and-a-half attempting this, they sure as heck weren't going to waste the results on me. But it didn't work, anyway.

Flat ironing back in my day was standing over an ironing board with the edge of your forehead barely touching that scratchy fabric liner. You'd have to stand there with your back and neck bent forward for as long as it would take. And if you had the thick hair that ran in our family, you could be there for a whole episode of *Dragnet.*

Well, my eldest sister went first because she had a dance to go to and she wanted to look nice. I waited patiently, watching my mother run her five-pound clothes iron over my other sisters' hair. Not all the kinks and curls disappeared, but they were less noticeable than before, and I couldn't wait to see my 'princess' hair again, instead of looking in the mirror at my puffed-up frizzy hair with little strands flying all over the place. A hundred plastic barrettes couldn't keep my hair tame, and I know because I tried.

By the time it was my turn, my mother was knee-deep in chores. She would iron a thin section of my hair, then run over to the stove to check on the cakes she was baking for our church bake sale, then check on my father because she had thought he'd said something from the den, but really he was just getting worked up about the nightly news. And then, after doing all that, she'd come back and iron another strand of my hair. If I attempted to move during any of this, my mother would smack my bottom with the giant wooden spoon she kept hanging on the wall for 'wasting her time,' so I didn't move an inch out of pure fear.

When the phone rang, my mother set down the iron, and I think she had every intention of attempting to finish my hair and stretch the corded phone over so she could gab at the same time, but my aunt was having another 'crisis' and my mom temporarily forgot about me. I smelled something burning before I felt any pain, but the time between the two was short. Before I knew it, my forehead and top of my scalp were on fire, and literally. My mother screamed and dropped the phone, and I'd never seen my dad move faster than he did that night. Dad grabbed the dishrag from the dirty dishwater and tossed it on my head like he was playing horseshoes.

I don't know what was more mortifying about this: the fact that only part of my waist-length hair burnt off and then burnt to my scalp, or that I had to go out in public with my hair looking like that until I could go to get the rest of it cut because the burns were irritated when I tried to wear a hat. I had to go through the rest of the school year without my long hair, and it took more than a year to get back to my original length just because my mom set the iron down on my hair while she went to answer the phone.

--N.S.

Then Indiana, now California

<u>That Was No Bird, Kevin</u>

I can tell you for a fact that the quickest medics you'll ever get are on their last run for the shift. This is relevant to this story because my partner and I were on our last run of a 24-hour shift, where we'd both probably gotten about four hours of sleep combined and we were ready to get the hell out of the station and go home. My partner had a wife who'd just had twins, so he was double-screwed and knew he wasn't going to be able to sleep at home, either, so I told him I'd drive and he could try to nap on the way to the scene, which was about fifteen minutes outside of town. We were responding to a three-car MVA.

It was raining and I was driving like a bat out of hell to this wreck. Cars ahead of me weren't getting out of the way and I think I picked up a bus chaser en route, so on top of being aggravated from no sleep, I was irritated with humanity. So when I got out of town I hit the gas a little harder and the last time I remember checking, we were flying down a two-lane country highway doing 70 MPH. I remember looking over to my partner, who'd already passed out with his lips smushed up against the window.

It was like a scene right out of a movie, I swear, because the very next thing I remember is seeing this car up ahead, coming my direction from the other lane, veering all over the place. It was dark and I really couldn't tell if the driver had hit something or was having a heart attack or was just drunk. I didn't have time to slow down before something huge flew at the truck and shattered the windshield.

My partner woke up doing some kind of weird karate thing with his hands and screamed, "Holy [crap], what kind of bird was that?"

The truck was in the process of skidding off the road and we ended up hitting a small tree, which brought us to a stop. Once we were able to get out, I realized how lucky we were. We had somehow avoided rolling down and over a steep hill on the side of the road. I think the truck's speed had a lot to do with essentially propelling us through the air until we landed.

"That was no bird, Kevin," I said too long later for it to be a properly-timed response.

He was still dazed and didn't know what was going on, so he asked, "What did you hit?"

We called in our predicament before walking back to the road and saw a doe lying in a pool of shattered glass from our windshield. There was a little bit of blood, too, and it wasn't moving. The car that was on the other side of the road had spun to a stop in what was my line moments before, and the front end was beat to trash. The driver was standing outside her door, calling 911. When she hit the deer, it was tossed in the air and went on a short flight until it smacked against our windshield.

Don't get all teary-eyed on me like my wife did. I swear, when I told her this story she was sobbing before I could tell her the 'happy ending.'

The deer took a few minutes to rest, apparently, right there in the middle of the road, before it stood up, surveyed her surroundings, and ran back to the woods.

We didn't have to go on the final run, which was a relief, but we had to go to the ER to be checked out before we could go home. Kevin told the nurses to take their time and he slept. I didn't have that option because I called my wife to let her know what happened and she rushed to the ER and talked for the whole three hours we were there.

That was the story of how my partner and I inspired a mandatory safety meeting at work and why there's now a recommendation for the secondary medic to be a deer lookout.

--T.S.
Ohio

The Unapproved Tenant

My team was called to a flat to respond to a geriatric chest pain complaint. We thought it would be a common scenario, but when we arrived there were groups of Bobbies (police) on scene, which had us rather apprehensive about entering the flat.

When we entered the flat, I was utterly flabbergasted that someone could live that way. There were piles of magazines stacked to my chest and dirty food wrappers scattered about the floor. It was only when a piece of rubbish caught on my boot and I attempted to kick it off was I able to see the flat's carpeting. I managed to kick up a sliver of rubbish to expose dirty burgundy carpet.

The smell inside of this flat was disgusting, and I mean it was so putrid that my partner had to step back into the hallway for to take a breather before we could respond to our patient, an elderly gent who I first assumed was in his mid-to-late 70s. He was instructed by other emergency responders to lie flat on the kitchen floor and had been given an aspirin to chew while waiting on our team.

My partner came in and we loaded the gent on the stretcher. The quickest and easiest route out of the flat was to travel back through the lounge (main sitting room), so the two of us worked on carrying the patient through the flat. My partner worked at the patient's feet and I at the patient's head.

As we moved to pass the sofa, I shouted and accidentally dropped my end of the stretcher. My partner could not hold the patient up alone, so his end went down as well, and the gent was moaning in pain from the fall, but I could not peel my eyes from what was on the sofa. That is the moment I realized why the Bobbies had responded to the flat as well.

On the sofa was a decaying corpse, sitting upright as if the deceased had passed while viewing the telly. Judging from the corpse's appearance, it had been left to decompose for a great deal of time. I could not quite make out the details of what the corpse would have looked like if he/she were still alive. Quite honestly, part of the only reason I knew it was even a human corpse was in large part of viewing bones and the hurrah taking place around me.

The elderly gent we were treating had allowed a transient to lodge with him some time ago. When the transient passed, the gent renting the flat was too scared to report it, fearing his flat owners would evict him for having an unapproved tenant. Instead, the elderly gent continued drinking heavily and left the lodger's body on the sofa.

My team was instructed not to discuss the incident with the press. My partner resigned shortly following the encounter. I have experienced night terrors regarding this call for several years but could never leave my employer because I love what I do.

--Submission details withheld at request
UK

Not in This Town

I work in a small town as an RN. We all know each other around here fairly well and most of us get along fine.

One night we were all cleaning and joshing around while the ER was empty (a rare occasion, as you know) when a call came in. The unit clerk was off making beds, and I was the closest one to her phone, so I answered and knew the voice on the other line right off the bat. It was one of my neighbors from across the street. Her sons snuck off to play and found their dad's drywall stilts. One son managed to 'strap in' the other son and the boy on the stilts staggered around the garage for a few seconds.

I could hardly understand my neighbor after that. I asked if she called for help, but I managed to comprehend that she did not, that her husband was on the way. She said something about 'all the blood' and hung up on me. I alerted the other three nurses on duty that we had an incoming patient to the ER entrance, and we took a bed outside to meet our patient.

We recognized the truck right away as one of dad's friends from work. Much to our surprise, dad was in the bed of the truck with his youngest son, a five-year-old. The stilts were still strapped to the boy's legs. The child was not breathing, and I could not make out the tiny features of his face that we'd all seen a million times before at church or the supermarket. It was the first time in my eight years on the job that I really felt afraid and lost. Things like this don't happen around here. We deal with complaints of coughs and colds and sometimes of broken arms or chest pain. I can't recall a time before this one of having a child under our care for an accident like this.

The boy's father was surprisingly calm for what he presented, and I'm positive he was in shock. He gave a report of what happened based off the story of the child's older brother, a seven-year-old. We didn't need the story, to be truthful, but the boy could not stand upright on the stilts, fell forward and hit his head on a beam, and then when he went down for real, he stretched his arms out to brace himself and landed face-first on the family's SUV's luggage rack. As if that wasn't bad enough, the boy rolled over, fell off the top of the SUV, and hit his head on the concrete floor.

We ran around like chickens with our heads cut off, trying to get this little man cleaned up and see exactly what we were looking at. Our unit clerk, bless her, knew from the story and commotion that we would need a flight team, so she called a children's hospital two hours away before we could get the blood wiped off his face.

In the end, it was determined the boy fractured both of his elbows, broke his right wrist, sustained a broken nose, knocked out two of his teeth, and suffered from a concussion. It was initially believed the boy had a hemorrhage of the spleen, but after a second opinion it appeared he only suffered minor bruising to the organ.

Our town pulled together to hold a cookout for the family's medical and travel expenses. The boy was released from the hospital a week after the accident. It was such a horrific ordeal that I would never wish upon even my worst enemy.

-M.P.

Texas

<u>Set Their Butts on Fire</u>

Back before I made Sheriff, I worked as an officer in a teeny-tiny town in West Virginia. I took the call from a woman I went to church with every Sunday. She was real upset, mad as a wet hen, really, because she caught our local troublemakers throwing bricks and stones through the windows of the church's old greenhouse. She was a little old lady who was afraid to go out and holler at the boys the whole town knew, so I told her to stay put and I'd come take care of it.

Those boys were trouble and a half, I swear on it. They were around 15 at the time and neither came from a real strong family environment, so they teamed up to terrorize the community and were always in trouble for something or another. This was back before the days of cellular phones or computers in every home, and where we lived there just wasn't much to keep good kids busy, so it wasn't much of a surprise that the bad apples were out causing grief so often.

When I pulled up to the greenhouse, neither of the boys ran. They never did. At least they had enough sense to know not to do that. Even if they ran, it's not like they had anywhere to go besides home.

Anyway, I hollered at the boys to hop in the back of my patrol car. I was going to take them home for the third time that week. They weren't scared at all. The one boy lived with his momma who worked all the time, and the other with his grandpa who was our local Otis, so they knew just as well as I did nothing was going to happen (again), and they'd be right back to it soon enough.

About five minutes into the ride home, I couldn't hear the boys over the sound of the radio anymore. I didn't think much of it until I smelled something burning. By the time I pulled over and got out of the car, the fire had spread over the whole backseat and the boys were laughing as my patrol car went up in flames. They'd used a hand lighter to set fire to the backseat.

Any goodness in my heart flew right away around that time. I snatched the boy nearest to me and flung him against the back of my burning car and tore into his hind end with my own belt. I don't know how many times I whipped him, but by the end he was crying and the other troublemaker was next. I whipped both of them until their butts were as hot as my vehicle.

The department wrote the car off as a loss and we eventually got a new one. I think back to that day and can't say I've ever lost my temper like that since then. Nowadays, doing that would land me on the news or in jail, but I'm confident it was what those two deserved and needed. I told them if I ever had to deal with them again they'd get it harder next time, and I never did get another call about them.

--K.Z.

West Virginia

Holla-Back Girl

My partner and I got dispatched to a 911 call for someone with their head stuck in a porch railing on Halloween.

When we rolled up to the sorority house I expected to see a bunch of drunk college kids all over the place, but it was like pulling up to a ghost town.

We walked up the sidewalk and could hear that Gwen Stefani song stuck on repeat during its course; it was blaring so loud I'm sure everyone in the area could hear it. There were empty red plastic cups and condoms and wrappers and beer cans all over the yard.

Up on the porch, we found the subject of the complaint. By the time we arrived on scene, she had passed out. She was on her knees, with her head stuck between the iron bars on the porch railing. She was also wearing one of those slutty costumes, but it was weird because I think she was supposed to be Elmo from *Sesame Street,* and it was the first time I'd ever seen someone try to pull off a sexy puppet Halloween costume.

While my partner and I were trying to pull the girl's head out from between the bars, one of her girlfriends ran out of the house wearing lingerie. One of her heels fell broke off her shoe as she was running around, screaming and crying, and she fell off the porch and said she needed to go to the hospital because she thought she broke her ankle.

So, at this point, to make sure we're together on this, we had one drunk girl passed out with her head stuck in a porch railing, and another drunk girl was rolling around on the sidewalk drunk-sobbing in a bra, panties, and lacy thigh-high nylons.

To make matters worse, we couldn't get the one girl's head maneuvered out from between the bars, so we called the station and requested the fire department. We were told the cops were en route because some of the neighbors called in a noise complaint, and dispatch thought the cops had tools we could use to remove the bars enclosing the girl's head.

While we were waiting for the cops, the drunk girl on the sidewalk freaked out and tried to run, but she really *did* break her ankle, so she went down again just as quickly as she did the first time. Her bra slipped, so now we had this drunk, hurt, crying, and *exposed* girl to tend to. While my partner was looking at her ankle, she told him everyone else had left when one of the neighbors said they called the cops, and she had to get out of there too because she was only 17. She lied to her friends and told them she was 22 so they'd let her drink, but I'm pretty sure most of the people there weren't 21, either, so…

Two officers showed up to the house a few minutes later and the girl on the sidewalk was still freaking out. It turns out it was for good reason because I guess her dad was on the force and the responding officers knew her. They pulled some strings and she got off the hook.

Now, the girl stuck in the porch railing was still our problem. We asked the cops if they had any tools with them to remove the bars from the railing, but nothing they had would work, so we had to ask dispatch (again) to call in the fire department, and then we had to wait for them to show up and cut the bars to free this girl.

When I pulled her away from the railing, she came to, said in a slur that she loved me, and then she vomited all down the front of my polo before passing out again. We transported her to the ER much to their displeasure—like I said, it was Halloween and they had been dealing with ETOH patients all night. I was able to sweet talk one of the techs into giving me an extra scrub top to wear until I could get back to the station and grab a clean shirt from my locker. I didn't want to walk around smelling like whiskey-puke until then.

The girl's BAC was three times the legal limit…well, for someone of age. We found out a little later that she, too, was underage. Shocker. The ER couldn't reach her parents but were able to reach a sibling. She was kept under observation for the night.

By the way, I freakin' hate working Halloween and I pray this one was my last because if not, next year I'm going to go crazy. Every single holiday is like this around here, but I'm pretty sure Halloween is the all-time worst.

  --A.B.
  Las Vegas, Nevada vicinity

Road Rage

I am a medic in a medium-sized city and have witnessed quite a bit of craziness, but the dumbest thing I've witnessed happened as I was staging (sitting in an ambulance parked in a strategically-chosen area to respond fastest to calls).

The intersection where I was staging was usually moderately busy, but on that day there wasn't much traffic, so I was blasting music and eating these brownies someone from the station made. I was bored out of my mind and had forgotten my cell in my jeans pocket, so until I could bribe someone to come out with my phone, I had nothing to do but people-watch.

Well, there I was, finishing up my last brownie when this big white van came speeding up to the four-way stop. It had to have been going at least 25 MPH and the driver didn't show any intention of stopping at his stop sign.

While I was more focused on the driver than anything else, the side door slid open and someone hopped out, did a roll on the ground, and then stood again. The van stopped.

I thought about calling this in because I wasn't sure what was going on, and with all these news stories about people getting kidnapped and stuff, I started to worry that was what I was seeing, like a reverse kidnapping.

As I picked up my radio to call it in, the person who'd jumped out of the van yelled something to the driver and the van started pulling forward again through the intersection, maybe going about half of the speed it was when the person jumped out.

I looked a little closer and realized the person who'd jumped out of the back of the van looked like a teen boy, and he was staggering a little as he started running toward the still-moving van.

"Why aren't these kids in school?" I muttered to myself, realizing I sounded more like my own parents than the rowdy kid I was in high school.

As I continued to watch, the boy attempted to dive back in the back of the van, but the driver sped up right as the boy took the leap. The teen hit the asphalt face-first and was screaming. There was blood all over his face. The driver of the van then *jumped out of the driver's seat as the van was still moving,* and the van crashed into a parked car on the other side of the intersection.

Now, the medic in me wanted to run over and help, but I can't. Nobody understands it, including me, but I am not supposed to respond to any scene without being dispatched to it.

I broke our company's rule and called over to the driver, another teen who'd run over to his injured friend, and I told him to call 911.

He said he couldn't because his parents would find out he and his friend had skipped school to steal from their liquor cabinet. He was more concerned with getting in trouble for that than he was getting his friend medical attention.

Thankfully, another witness called in the accident and I was dispatched to the scene.

The first van-jumper broke his jaw when he tried to jump back in the van. His friend sprained his ankle when he hopped from the driver's seat.

I read in the paper that damage to the *brand new* parked *sports car* was over $3,000. Both teens were drunk.

--J.B.

New York

Christmas Birthday

I saw the picture you posted on Twitter (posted by a satirical group with the text, 'The upcoming holidays are not medical reasons for labor induction.'), and it immediately brought back memories of this occurring a few years ago.

I was working on OB as a nurse's assistant when a woman was wheeled upstairs by our orderly. She wasn't due until March, which put her right around the late sixth-early seventh-month mark, and she wasn't having contractions. When I heard a nurse ask politely what her problems were, the woman replied her problem was that she wasn't in labor and Christmas was two days away. The mother went on and on about how much she wanted to have a Christmas baby, especially because her sister-in-law was also due in March, and if she couldn't have this baby now, she'd never 'get any of the attention [she] deserves.'

Boy, oh boy, were my eyes wide open. After I picked up my jaw from the floor, I hurried away and kind of lingered at the end of the hall. I wanted to hear what the nurse was going to say back to the woman, but I didn't want my shock to be obvious and get reported.

As expected, the RN stated the hospital would be glad to treat the patient for any pain she was experiencing and address any concerns she had for her child's wellbeing, but they adamantly refused to induce labor for the sake of the child having a Christmas birthday. The woman was upset and called for a ride home.

I came back three days later and the patient was the talk of the floor. She had been brought in to the ER because she had attempted to induce labor 'naturally' by doing things she found on the internet (she attempted acupuncture on herself, for one, and I was told she drank a significant amount of castor oil), and once her family discovered what she was doing, they felt it best to bring in the patient for a psychiatric evaluation. Our counselors must have agreed that this woman was a danger to not only herself but to her unborn child, and they placed her in an emergency treatment room. She was brought to our floor on the second night because she had taken to jumping up and down on her bed to 'get the baby out,' and then she complained the baby stopped moving.

From what my coworkers told me, the baby was fine but the mother was crying and begging them to take the baby out of her so he/she could have that Christmas birthday.

I don't know whatever happened to that woman or her child, but I can tell you for a fact that these things happen—as crazy and wild as the stories sound to others.

--S.P.

Rhode Island

<u>Oops</u>

I work in lab services and three years ago the police department's regular lab was shut down after a fire, so they rerouted all of their blood and urine tests for us. This meant we were swamped, buried up to our eyeballs in tests for DUIs, parole violations, and weekly probation tests, all on top of our regular OP and IP tests we had to administer. Much like your department, we didn't get a lot of extra help, so we were all overwhelmed and overworked, and I just couldn't wait for it to all be over with.

One day a young man came in and said he was there for his probation urine test. Usually, we ask everyone to empty his/her pockets, step behind a curtain, and urinate in a cup. Females are given a 'potty chair,' but are asked to complete the process just the same. Once the process is complete, the patient will place the cup on a shelf and go to the washroom to wash his/her hands. We then test the urine for traces of illegal substances.

Because, like I said, we were swamped, our 'pee booths' were full. I sent the man to the washroom just so I could get him out of there quicker, and I thought the process went smoothly. He returned his cup of urine to my 'pee shelf,' and then returned to the washroom to clean up. I sent him to our waiting room outside of our office and he pulled out a cell phone and started playing games or texting or whatever he was doing.

I ran the first test and when I saw the results, I scolded myself for getting confused and mixing up patients. But when I tested his urine a second time, I knew I had to call in the results to the police department.

The man came back to my window twice to ask if I could sign his release form so he could go, but I had to lie and tell him I was so busy that it was going to take longer than usual, even though I had already managed to release five other patients in that time. He seemed nervous.

When the officers arrived, I explained that the patient's urine yielded a positive pregnancy test, as well as traces of methamphetamines and THC. When confronted, the patient broke down and said he smoked pot and was afraid of being busted for it, so he asked his girlfriend to urinate in a Ziploc bag for him and he had hidden the baggy inside his waistband. He stated he did not know his girlfriend was pregnant, nor did he know she was participating in meth usage. He did know she smoked pot because they did it together routinely, but he said he didn't know she still had it in her system because the 'plan' was for her to stay clean so he could test clean and get off probation. Then, they would go back to partying together.

For a minute, I felt really bad for the patient. Then three more patients came in and I guess I got over it.

Moral of my story: if you're going to get someone to pee for you, make sure they're clean too. Oh, and make sure they're not pregnant.

--L.J.
Michigan

No Faith in Humanity

I'll keep this short but not so sweet.

I'm a PA-C in an ER inside a high-traffic metropolitan trauma center. We see things that I won't even try to describe because they still make me sick, and I'm a combat veteran. That's saying something.

One night, a patient was transported for a GSW (gunshot wound) to the left temple, sustained during a robbery. Remarkably, the patient was very much alive (the bullet was fired from a distance; if it had not been the patient would have been DOA) and communicative. He actively refused any form of sedation or medications that would render him unable to communicate with his family. This man stated he knew he was going to die, and he wanted to see his wife first. Only then would he accept drugs. I attempted multiple times, until I was blue in the face, to explain to the patient that the bullet was positioned in such a way that he was barely hanging on and waiting was not an option for his health. Still, he refused all options and demanded nothing be done until his wife arrived.

I cannot imagine this man's excruciating pain. As the minutes passed, he took to screaming loudly and moaning. I must admit that I agreed with the patient's self-diagnosis: he was likely to die, with the bullet's positioning. I discussed the patient with the trauma surgeon and other ER physicians, as well as the nurses; we all agreed to allow the patient to choose his own treatment plan until his wife arrived.

I returned to my desk to overlook my next patient's chart and was rudely interrupted by a middle-aged woman from the room located next to the GSW.

"My husband hurt his foot and nobody's been in to see him. When is someone coming to see him?"

Lo and behold, after asking the patient's name, I realized I was holding his chart and he was next in line.

"And can you do something to shut that guy up?" the woman asked, with saliva flying out of her mouth as she spoke. She nodded toward the GSW room. "He's annoying as hell."

Without violating HIPAA, I explained the patient was suffering from a serious wound, but she wouldn't hear it.

"And I have a headache," she retorted. "I don't care what his problem is. Just shut him up."

The GSW victim did not live long enough to see his wife.

--T.F.W.
Los Angeles, California vicinity

Get This Woman a Calendar

Kerry, true story here.

I'm an OB-GYN on call for the ER and by coincidence happened to be in the ER when a woman was transported via EMS for abdominal pain and bleeding in early pregnancy. The RNs were drowning in patients presenting with cold and flu symptoms, so I (rather stupidly) volunteered myself to oversee the most recent OB complainant.

The meeting was average. I listened as the patient explained she was six-weeks pregnant with twins, and I explained to her that abdominal pain and cramping throughout pregnancy is quite normal. She expressed concerns about vaginal bleeding, so I completed a vaginal exam and found no signs of bleeding. Together, we concluded she was probably spotting. Again, I assured her this was normal within the early pregnancy period.

The patient then asked if I would complete an ultrasound, and just to ease her mind, I said I would.

Something struck me as odd.

"It would appear that you are much farther along than six weeks," I commented.

"No," she argued, becoming defensive almost immediately.

I pointed to several points on the screen and attempted to rationalize the fetuses' measurements.

"I'm six weeks," the patient said again. "I went to a doctor a month ago and she told me."

Now, in my field I've heard a similar story repeated as a joke, but I must admit the joke must have started after another physician experienced a similar patient. I still am having trouble processing that this woman will be a mother in a few months.

--G.J.P.

Florida

Well, That IS a Valid Reason

I work as a secretary in an Orthopedic clinic and because we are located in the heart of our county, surrounded by smaller villages but still hundreds of miles away from larger cities, we have to screen and prioritize our patients' visits and surgeries by not only what the surgeon believes to be necessary procedures, but patient 'determination' as well. For example, if you come in for joint pain and are told to first lose weight, but you flat-out refuse a change in your diet and/or exercise regiment, it's my job to place you after a patient willing to adhere to the doctor's suggestion(s).

This makes for a difficult job, just because patients often become angry with me that they have to wait. Some of our waiting times for surgeries or rehab are a year-long.

My favorite story about my job is the time we had to evaluate an elderly man's placement on a hip surgery list. Yes, he was in pain, but he retained mobility.

He was booking his next appointment with me and asked if he could have his surgery moved up.

I asked, "Sir, what reason do you have to believe your surgery should come before our other patients' surgeries?"

This 80-something-year-old man leaned in, looked me square in the eyes, and said without missing a beat, "Because I want to have more sex before I die, and I can't do it with a bum hip."

Our surgeon thought the man's excuse was not only humorous but also a good one, and we scheduled the patient for surgery the following week.

--B.R.

Iowa

At Least He Was Trying

N.P. (Nurse Practitioner) here. I work in a small office with only a handful of rooms and not much staff. We operate out of a moderately-populated town.

I once had a patient come to me with off-the-chart cholesterol and triglyceride levels. The patient was medically classified as 'morbidly obese,' with a height around 5'8" and a weight around 350 pounds.

Naturally, I explained kindly to the patient that his weight and cholesterol levels were far from ideal. I asked if he would be willing to try a new diet for me, to which he agreed. We went over how important vegetables were to a healthy diet, discussed cutting out sugary soft drinks, and compromised on a healthy amount of 'starter' exercise.

A month later, when I saw the patient again, he had gained more than *twenty* pounds.

"I don't understand," he told me. "I've been eating five servings of vegetables every day, and I stopped drinking soda."

I asked the patient if he'd been working out, to which he responded he had. The patient said he'd started meeting with a group of women in his subdivision to walk a few blocks each night. This upset him even more, as he felt he was 'wasting his life, since nothing else he was doing mattered.'

I was at loss at what to do, so I asked the patient if he would feel comfortable keeping a food journal for me. In this journal/notebook, he would log each and every food/drink he consumed over the course of a week, and then he would bring it back to me. The log was to contain either a precise or estimated portion of the food he was consuming, the time of consumption, and his mood during the time of consumption. I chose to add the latter because my patients often confess to 'emotional eating,' where they consume foods based on depression or boredom, rather than hunger. If we could narrow down a specific time or mood or ingredient to which the patient was attracted, I thought perhaps we could alter his diet further.

After a week, my patient returned. During his weigh-in, we realized he had gained another three pounds! I asked him to come to my office so I could look over his food journal with him by my side, should I have any questions, and he followed me to my cramped office.

At first glance, I suppose I was dismayed at the patient's choice in meals during his first day. For breakfast he consumed three frozen breakfast burritos, two glasses of orange juice, and then he finished off the meal with a tube of yogurt. None of these items were what I would consider 'healthy.' The microwave burritos alone exceeded his sodium needs for the entire day; the orange juice was packed full of sugar; and the yogurt was full of sugar and artificial flavoring.

Lunch for the patient consisted of a 'low-cal' option from a local restaurant, that still packed in the pounds at 600 calories. The patient added he drank sweetened ice tea and ate three rolls, sans butter.

For dinner, the patient logged he consumed a large pizza from [a well-known pizza joint]. He ordered a spinach and feta topping on hand-tossed crust.

Okay, maybe that was a 'cheat day.'

When I looked over the patient's exercise log and dessert, I realized something.

"So you walk with women from your subdivision each night after supper?"

He nodded.

"Just around the block?" I asked.

He shook his head. "No. We go for ice cream."

That would explain the large hot fudge sundaes he logged each night.

Throughout the rest of the week, the patient did appear to be trying on a consistent basis. He began swapping sweet tea and juice for water sporadically throughout the day, and occasionally he would order a salad from a fast food joint. This still isn't the best option, but he was *trying.* I scolded him on how many cheesy potatoes he consumed and discussed how starch is processed by the body, and we tried to come up with other vegetables he could consume with cheese, that would not be the ideal food on my menu, but would ease him in to eating more veggies.

Each day of the menu, however, disappointed me and explained exactly why the patient was gaining weight instead of losing it. Every single night, the patient consumed a large pizza topped with spinach and feta cheese. According to the company's nutritional pamphlet, the crust alone is slightly over 1400 calories. In addition, the sauce on the pizza comes in at a little over 500 calories; the cheese adds another 550-ish calories; and the spinach adds 15. Each night, the patient was consuming nearly 2,500 calories *before* beverages, dipping sauces, side dishes, or desserts. Every other night, the patient would order a chocolate dessert that contained close to 600 calories…and then take his 'walk' for ice cream with the neighborhood women.

When I pointed this out to the patient he looked at me with a dumbfounded expression and said, "I thought it was okay because you said I needed vegetables in my diet, so I ordered spinach as a topping instead of meat."

I learned from this patient the need for nutritional education. I'm no Skinny Sam myself, and it's okay to indulge (I love my weekend wine and churros!), but many people are simply choosing the wrong foods, oblivious to what those foods do to the body.

Good news, though: my patient did lose 100 pounds through diet and exercise. He still enjoys his hot fudge sundae each night.

--A.K.

Kentucky

<u>Miracle</u>

The worst and best night I have ever experienced in my entire career as an ER RN happened on the same night, with the same patient.

A call came over that a toddler was found unresponsive after falling in a neighbor's pool. Nobody knew how long the child had been in the water, but EMS reported the family realized the girl was missing and narrowed down the time she was gone to be between 15 and 20 minutes. Unfortunately, it only takes a fraction of that time for a child to drown.

The child had a pulse at the time she was removed from the pool, and EMS was escorted by nearby patrol cars. The police department actually closed down major intersections to allow the medics to transport the patient as quickly as possible.

Rather than pull up in the ambulance bay, the medics stopped in front of the ER and one of the medics—a father himself—carried the child inside. The ER lobby was already full. Some of the people there were injured. Some were feeling under the weather. Some, honestly, we saw every single day and I wanted to tell them to go back home instead of standing in the way, staring, as this medic tried to save this child's life. I've never hated patients more than I did in that moment. Even now, I think back to that moment, when all of these people were just *standing* there, complaining about the wait times, making jokes about getting the day off from work, crying about how it wasn't *fair* that EMS was allowed to bring in a patient in front of all the patients who'd been waiting…my heart fills with this incomprehensible, indescribable *rage*.

I pointed the medic to a trauma bay and he situated the toddler on the bed. She was so tiny, pale, fragile. Her blonde hair was still wet and matted to the side of her thin cheek. Her fingernails were painted bright pink, to match her romper. She only had one sandal on.

And her heart wasn't beating anymore.

The medic stated the child's heart stopped as the truck pulled onto hospital property.

I continued with chest compressions and heard blood-curdling screaming from the hallway. The patient's mother had arrived and was blaming herself for her child wandering off during a barbecue. Fear and shame took over. I had to save this baby. Not saving her was not an option. In that moment, if I could have taken my own life to allow her to take another breath, I gladly would have done it without a second thought. Nursing school didn't prepare me for this. Hell, actually working in the ER didn't prepare me for this. Nothing can ready you for what you see here. Nothing.

I began sobbing so hard during the process that two of my coworkers pulled me from the child's side and escorted me out of the room and to the back hallway, out of the mother's sight. Though my ears were ringing and I couldn't breathe through all the snot plugging up my nose, though I couldn't see through the tears and I regretted wearing eyeliner that day because it had melted into my eyes, which made them burn even more…I could still hear the patient's mother screaming. I *still* hear the patient's mother screaming sometimes, along with all the other families of patients we've lost over the years I've worked there.

That's something they don't tell you. They don't tell you in nursing school that you'll see these people in your dreams or that you'll have to live with yourself after you deliver the news of death, or that you'll never be able to forget the sounds of the shrieking the mother of a teen MVA victim did when she pushed by a line of nurses trying to prevent her from seeing that her daughter's head was nearly decapitated. It's all unsaid. You're supposed to just *know* that you'll deal with these things, and you're just supposed to *know* how to deal with it. And you're supposed to just *move on*, maybe not so much forget what's occurred by don't let it be part of who you are as a person, who you are as a nurse.

That's bullshit. You have to let these things join you as a nurse willingly or they take you, anyway. And you do bounce back. You do move on. You use that fear, those emotions, while you're working on a patient.

You show those emotions to share the family's burden, to let them know they're not alone.

The little girl was pronounced dead, and your books are accurate in describing the ER after a death, especially that of a child. We were quiet. There were other patients to treat, but it wasn't the same. The smiles were forced. We were all intolerant of the complaints about how we were out of Diet Coke for family members or how the cafeteria was closed or that someone actually had to *wait* fifteen minutes in an *emergency* room.

The drowning victim's family went in the room to stay with her until the coroner arrived. We closed the curtain to give them privacy.

Eleven minutes later, we all heard frantic shouting from the room and I think I may have jumped over two rolling desk chairs to make it to the room first. When we pulled back the curtain, the patient's mother had lifted the child to a sitting position and was holding her tightly. The patient's father was on his knees, sobbing.

And the toddler's eyes were open.

She was *alive.*

The little girl was rushed to our peds ICU wing and was on a respirator for close to a week, but she was released in good condition after another week of observation.

I don't know what happened in that room. I don't know what happened with that child's life in the hands of God. But I can tell you from experience that miracles *do* happen. Sometimes you're lucky enough to see one happen right in front of your eyes.

--M.C.

Mississippi

<u>For Better or Worse</u>

The absolute worst patient I've ever encountered was transported by ambulance…while she was still wearing her wedding gown.

Medics wheeled in an obscenity-shouting woman flailing on the stretcher to the point that she nearly tipped herself over as the team attempted to transport the patient to a non-trauma room. She consumed a little (okay, a *lot*) too much to drink at her own open bar, and when her family arrived, the patient's mother explained the patient had already become a little rowdy with the first few drinks. But when her groom's (pregnant) ex-girlfriend arrived (unannounced) at the reception venue, the drunken bride became violent. She allegedly attacked the ex-girlfriend, breaking glasses, chairs, and collapsing tables in the process.

Dear Lord, was this woman a complete nightmare. She repeatedly spit on staff, had no loss of words when it came to insulting all of us, and she urinated all over her dress and bed and then threatened to sue the hospital over her gown's ruined condition.

The patient had deep lacerations on her arm and shoulder from the ex-girlfriend slicing her open with a broken wine glass. After 20 minutes of fighting, she finally allowed me to clean her up, suture some of the wounds, and bandage the rest. Then, though, as I was packing up my suture kit, she ripped the bandages off her wounds and started tearing the sutures out of her skin.

I reported this behavior to one of the doctors and was told to restrain the patient with cuffs, then call our mental health on-call counselor for a consultation.

Restraining this woman was worse than trying to change the diaper on a screaming, kicking baby. I ride bulls as a hobby and would rather have been on one then than trying to restrain this piece of work. She punched me twice and I had to walk away to keep myself from choking her to death. I called for help and it took three security guards, a tech, and another nurse to get the woman cuffed to the bed rails.

To make matters worse, someone from up front let the patient's mother come back, and then the mom started taking pictures with her cell phone. She was screaming at everyone, saying she was going to sue the hospital for 'inhumane' treatment. We tried to keep her out of the room, but she went in there and *removed the restraints* from her daughter.

When this happened, the doctor told the unit clerk to call the police.

While we were waiting for the police to show up, the patient's mother helped her out of bed and the two made their way to the lobby.

Out in the lobby were the patient's new husband, the ex-girlfriend, and about half of her wedding party. They weren't fighting until the patient and her mother went out there, but as soon as the ex-girlfriend and the bride saw each other, the fight was on again.

Innocent patients were caught up in the squabble, and security tried to separate everyone. One woman was registering for a labor check, when the bride dove at the ex-girlfriend—who moved at the last moment—

and the bride knocked the registering patient to the floor. The registration people were freaking out, patients in the waiting room were screaming, most of the wedding party had become involved in the brawl, and the husband had taken to trying to protect his ex from his new wife.

When the police arrived, almost everyone stopped fighting. The bride was still on a rampage and was in the process of thrusting a wheelchair across the lobby at the time she was brought down with a taser. She still tried to fight as she was flopping around on the floor, and the ex-girlfriend was still going after her. The ex managed to get one last kick to the bride's face before an officer yanked her away and put her in cuffs.

Almost everyone from the patient's visiting pool was arrested. We had to medically clear the bride for jail, but by that time we were *done* with her shenanigans, so the doctor did a quick once-over and declared her fit for incarceration.

The incident made the local paper, but I didn't see the bride again. I did, however, see the groom, with his new wife (the ex), when she came in to have their baby.

Holy crap. Just…holy crap.

--Z.R.

Georgia

Wait Until You Hear the Worst Part

I work registration, too, but I think our hospital is bigger than yours. I've only done the job for a year, but the end of my first week was probably the worst day I've had yet.

I knew the system from filing and working patient accounts at another hospital, so the computer wasn't an issue for me. On the first day I was already registering people. We don't do what you do, though. At this hospital, we register patients for complaints, move them to booths, and collect information. If they have major issues, a nurse brings them to our booths when they're discharged, or they'll send a family member. The *only* time I have to go to a room is when the patient doesn't have family, isn't being discharged, or can't come to our booth (like an elderly person going back to the nursing home).

A guy came in with his kid and he was having an allergic reaction, so he had to go straight back to a room. Naturally, his kid went with him.

Well, a nurse told me the patient didn't have family coming, so I had to go to his room to get contact and insurance information. No big deal. I have a little tablet that I take to the back, so the process doesn't take too long. The patients can even use a stylus to sign e-forms for consent, so it's a pretty easy, in-and-out thing.

The patient was very nice to me. His pre-teen daughter? Not so much.

"Go get me a Diet Pepsi," she snapped at me, as I was saying goodbye to her father.

I wanted to roll my eyes and leave, but instead told her, "I'm sorry, but we don't have pop available for patients or families. I can have someone show you to the snack shop, if you'd like."

If I had to describe her transformation, I'd say it was like Satan spawning from Hell.

This girl stood from her chair, got in my face, cursed at me, and told me again to bring her a pop. I looked to her father for help, but he just shrugged and said, "She's thirsty."

"We don't have pop available for patients or families," I said again. This time I wasn't as polite with my deliverance, but I didn't give a care in the world.

I tried to walk out, and that's when I felt something hit the center of my knees. I fell to the ground. The patient's daughter had picked up her chair and hit me with it.

I called out for help and a nurse ran to the room. As he was helping me up, the patient's daughter dropped her pants and underwear, and then she defecated on the floor.

All the patient had to say for his daughter is that she 'has a hard time hearing the word no' and he made no apology for her behavior.

The worst part of all of this *wasn't* that there was nothing we could do. The patient didn't have family to come get his [bad word] of a child, she couldn't be prosecuted or removed from hospital property because she was underage and her only legal guardian was a patient. Oh, and I had to go back in the room twice…once to tell the patient his insurance came back invalid and another time to give him a complaint form because he 'didn't like my attitude.' Nope. The worst part of all of this is that, despite two nurses backing my story *and* verifying that I was never rude to the patient or his evil kid, I was written up for inappropriate attitude toward a patient and/or family of a patient. Then, a month later, at my probationary eval, my boss told me since I had that complaint filed against me, I was ineligible for a raise and told me I was lucky she didn't can me in the first place.

Luckily, that boss was fired and I never saw that patient (or his daughter, especially) again.

--M.P.
North Dakota

One of Our Own

Your story about how one of your nurses was killed by a drunk driver tugged at my heartstrings because our ER experienced something similar.

We had an inmate brought in one night from a maximum-security prison not too far from us. The guy was a real piece of work, spitting on everyone and cursing. He was experiencing tachycardia per his complaint, so we went to hook him up to the EKG lines and he went berserk, attacking a female tech and trying to get her in bed with him. Security rushed to the room to help the corrections guard with an emergency restraint, but the patient somehow kicked our security guard in the head, knocking him unconscious.

The patient was restrained and we moved the security guard to another room and registered him. We were hoping he was just knocked out and would have a minor concussion, but it turned out the inmate kicked the guard so hard he experienced a brain bleed and died shortly after the incident.

To say it was difficult to care for this jerk after he killed one of our guards is an understatement. Everyone in the building hated the man and people were walking around crying and were forced to put aside their emotions to treat other patients. Administration called in crisis counselors from another hospital, since we don't have a unit, and the counselors were taking our staff to consult rooms, the chapel, and basically anyplace there was room to have a session.

Someone called the security guard's family and when his wife showed up with the couple's adult children, I couldn't contain my emotions. The man who'd killed a husband, father, grandfather (so on) was still a patient and was located three rooms away from our security guard's body. And you know what was sick about the whole thing? He could hear everyone crying and he was screaming loudly, bragging about what he did, laughing about killing a 'cop.'

We had to treat this piece of scum like we'd treat any other patient, when all we really wanted to do was take him out.

The inmate was admitted to the ICU floor and had to go in for an emergency bypass in the middle of the night. I know it's wrong to say, but I was hoping the surgeon would accidentally clip an artery or something.

--T.E.

Florida

<u>Your Options</u>

I'm just going to start off by saying I'm a black man and I'm gay and I'm kind of feminine with my mannerisms and how I talk. My fellow RNs are awesome and we love each other, and I have never been made to feel left out or discriminated against by any of the ER nurses.

Now patients are a different story.

I get called all kinds of names by patients when they're mad they can't get a fix or they think ten minutes is too long to wait when I've been in the next room trying to start a central line. I usually just let it roll right off my shoulders because my grandmother always told me that hate usually stems from jealousy, so I just like to imagine all these hateful, inpatient people just wish they could have my figure or my clear complexion.

There was one evening shift that I was just not in any good mood. I was scheduled from 5A-5P, but someone called in on an already short-staffed shift, so I was told I had to stay until 9P. It was about 19:00 (7 PM) and I hadn't eaten since about noon, and girl let me just tell you my body ain't built that way. The Good Lord knew when he made me I need Little Debbie in my life at least every other hour. At this point, I was close to chewing my own arm off.

I finally got everything caught up and had a minute to run to the restroom *and* grab something to snack on, but right as I was sitting down to eat a sandwich I found in the break room fridge, one of the girls up front ran to the back all red-faced and screamed that she thought a patient was having a heart attack in the lobby. Charge sent me up front and I didn't even get to take one bite of that sandwich.

When I got to the lobby this woman, probably in her mid-40s, was lying on the dirty floor, clutching her chest. She was screaming words my grandmother would have slapped my lips off for saying, announcing to everyone she was having a heart attack and that nobody was helping her. Drama queen of the year would have easily gone to that woman if we had an awards ceremony for the ER.

"Ma'am," I said calmly, "we're gonna need to get you in a wheelchair and we're gonna go back to a room right away, okay?"

And you know what this lady had the nerve to say to me? This tubby roly-poly, two-thousand-dollar-necklace around her neck, diamond rings on every finger, tennis-skirt-wearing lady told me she wasn't going anywhere with a [homosexual n-word].

So, because I am such a well-mannered professional nurse, I said to her, "Fine, then. You can just lay right on our floor and die if you want to."

Her heart attack must have taken a pause because she jumped right up from that floor and demanded to see someone in charge to make a complaint.

The issue with this was we're in the middle of Atlanta and this witch wanted to only speak to someone of her color, so when the black charge nurse came out to the lobby, the woman went off again, throwing around the n-word like she was talking about a Kohl's sale or something. I wish I could believe she didn't know how she was making herself look or how she was making others feel, but I have a feeling that she used the word frequently and on a daily basis.

We didn't have a Caucasian nurse available to take on another patient, so this woman was told by the charge that if she wanted care she would have to be seen by a black nurse.

The woman refused but wouldn't leave. She was causing a big scene by going to the waiting room and yelling that her rights were being violated and this and that and anything she could say just to rile people up. Most of the people in the waiting room were also black and were becoming agitated.

One of the girls up front paged security to the waiting room and our two (black) guards tried to escort the woman off the property after giving her one more chance to register as a patient.

And you know what this crazy woman did? She pulled out pepper spray from her purse and sprayed the guards!

Someone called 911 while we tried to restrain the woman. She was shouting the n-word nonstop and screaming that we were trying to kill her.

In the end, she did get to speak to a white person in charge: her arresting officer.

The guards had to go to our decontamination room and then were relieved of duty for the night. I went right back to my desk and ate my sandwich like nothing ever happened.

It wasn't even a full moon. It was just a normal Thursday.

--J.R.

Georgia

<u>Replying to a Tweet</u>

Hey, I started following your Twitter and saw that you tweeted about some of the chaos after the Cubs won the Series. It was especially funny to me because I live in Cleveland and work in the ER, and my best friend since grade school works in the ER in Chicago. We made a lot of jokes because we both hate each other's teams, but it was all in good fun.

Anyway, I asked my friend about the people climbing poles around the stadium and she said they received *tons* of patients with fall complaints just from climbing the poles. Most were lucky and suffered from minor abrasions, some fractures. I do know she said one patient hit his/her head during the fall and it was touch-and-go there for a while. (I'm afraid to give more details at risk of getting my friend in trouble, so I do hope you'll excuse my candidness. *Quick author's note: Never apologize for protecting your patients, for one. Two, all stories have been edited, several times over if there is a request. Three, I'm happy to have you as a reader/follower and am thrilled to hear from you!)

What really didn't surprise me when we were catching up on the game and working after the game, was that she also treated a lot of GSWs and she said EMS and LEOs even responded to explosions.

Cleveland was a little worse off than usual, but I can't say we had too many outrageous cases. I do recall that we saw a handful of suicide attempts/ideations shortly following the game results. We handled slightly more ETOH patients than we did during the last Super Bowl. Most of the ETOH patients were sore losers and kept to themselves while they were vomiting or crying, but one man was brought in for a medical jail clearance and he had to be stripped by security and cops because he pulled a knife out of his underwear while the doctor was examining him.

The craziest thing I saw all night wasn't that crazy for our ER. A patient was brought in by medics with a broken beer bottle protruding from his/her back. According to the patient, he/she was involved in a bar fight, the other person broke a beer bottle & shoved it in his/her back, and then the fight was over.

I'm sorry I couldn't tell you more, but you know how it goes in this business!

--Anonymous at request

Ohio

<u>The Bad Parent(s) Club</u>

I have received many submissions regarding neglectful, abusive, or silly parenting from readers. Here are just a few:

*

I called Child Services when my patient was brought in unresponsive. She was two. Her dad thought it would be funny to see how much alcohol she could drink. He said he gave her two and a half small cans of a strawberry malt drink. She nearly died and had to be transferred to a specialist once she was stabilized for transport. I actively followed this case and almost lost my job when the hospital found out I was contacting CPS and the family for updates, but I am happy to report the child's mother now has full custody and the girl's father is still in jail on several charges.

--B.L.

South Carolina

*

The worst thing I've ever seen while working here is a kid mauled by pit bulls. I have nothing against the breed because I have two and they're great with my family's kids. (Please make sure to put that if you use my story because I don't want people continuing the hatred against the breed.)

I think the nurses said the patient was two or three. Her P.O.S parents used her as bait in their dog fighting ring because they said using the girl worked up the dogs better than animals did. I guess they'd been doing this for a while, and when the fight would start someone would take the girl out of the ring and let the dogs fight.

Whatever the case was, the girl was covered in blood and there was blood all over the trauma room. My department was responsible for cleaning the room and it took so long to get all the blood out of there that we had to put the room on a block for my entire shift. There was just so much blood and we kept finding it, even after we'd cleaned a million times.

I heard the girl didn't die, but she had to get her arm amputated and had more than 100 stitches. Please don't use my name or where I'm from because the parents are from a bad group and I don't want to get targeted for telling the story.

*

A new mom brought her newborn back to the hospital two days after discharge and said she thought there was something wrong with him because she read on the internet that babies didn't poop until they were at least a month old.

--M.N.
North Carolina

*

So, I've read all of your books and the only story I have to compete is that one time this lady brought her newborn in with chemical burns to its head and patches of hair either missing or seared off because mom didn't like all the baby's hair and used Nair to get it off.

--C.K.

Oregon

*

Four-year-old was brought in on my shift because she set herself on fire while trying to make herself lunch, after seeing her 'mother' make lunch for *herself*, but not the child.

The kid told the counselors that her mom didn't cook meals and her meals consisted of cookies, crackers, and eating dry ramen noodles from the pack (when she could get them open).

My spouse was the case counselor for this child and said when family members were interviewed they all backed up the kid's story. If mom fed the kid at all, she pretty much picked up a bag of chips from the store and that was the kid's lunch and dinner. Mom also slept all day and let her kid run around naked. The kid didn't have a bed and there were roaches and dog feces on her bedroom floor. Oh, and mom thought it was okay to leave the kid at home while she went out to eat or to see a movie with whichever boyfriend she was seeing.

--J.D.G.
Illinois

*

Eight years ago, I responded to a call of a crying baby and thought it was going to be some nosy neighbor complaint.

I repeatedly knocked on the door for several minutes before calling in to dispatch to find out more about the complainant. It was a neighbor, who told me she heard the door close the day before and only heard a crying baby since. No other officers had responded to the calls, according to the neighbor of the adjoining duplex.

I called in again reasonable suspicion to enter and received backup to forcefully enter the apartment. All I could smell when I opened the door was feces. I followed the smell to the room where the crying child was lying in a crib. The baby had filled her diaper and the diaper had exploded.

Being a father myself, I wanted to pick up the baby and give her a bath and feed her, but we had to wait to take photographs of the neglect.

The entire situation had me livid. The baby wasn't even old enough to roll over or hold her own bottle, though there was one filled with spoiled formula in the room with her.

We tracked the baby's mom down at a boyfriend's house. She was on a cocaine binge while her baby was alone for what we could estimate (based on the neighbor's testimony) to be about 26 hours.

After fantastic work by DCFS, my department, and the neighbor, I am proud to say I was eventually approved to foster the baby and my wife and I officially adopted her on her first birthday.

--J.P.
Nevada

*

I don't even know how many times I've had to explain to parents that *farting* does not mean the child is allergic to a food.

--D.R.
Delaware

Scanner Feed

This is one of my own little tidbits to add to the book. I still listen to the scanner and this is what I've been hearing in the days leading up to the full moon:

- Officers dispatched to a residence after a female complained of witnessing her neighbors urinating on stray cats

- Four structure fires in two days, resulting in total loss in each case

- Officers dispatched to break up a fight between two female adults. Not much information was given during the scanner feed, but I was able to hop on one of our community Facebook pages and witness the online fight that resulted in a real life, physical altercation. The fight seemed to stem from one of the women calling the other a 'dirty skank' and alleging drug abuse.

- Several concerned citizens contacted the police department after seeing a grown man dressed as a baby walking down the street at three in the morning, but officers were unable to locate the subject.

- Angry after receiving a nuisance ticket, a woman rammed her car into a squad car. She was immediately arrested and was booked on drug charges in addition to the MVA charges.

- BOLO (be on lookout) issued for two individuals robbing adjacent county liquor stores—the subjects were described as wearing Halloween costumes. One was dressed as the knifeman from *Scream* and the other was dressed as a clown, wearing full makeup.

- Officer requested in response to assault charges—a man dressed as a clown stated he was 'just trying to scare' people in the Wal Mart parking lot and wished to file assault charges against a woman who maced him. Clown subject was arrested on outstanding warrants.

- Dispatch received complaints regarding a fast-moving vehicle on the highway tossing live animals out of the passenger window. Three live puppies, approximately five weeks old, were recovered, one with critical injuries.

Public Service Announcement

I do so hope you will share this because it is clear our youth can't comprehend the severity of their actions, and I am not so sure parents are aware of what their children are doing when they are not being monitored correctly.

I have been in Emergency Services for 23 years and have seen my fair share of stupid patients, but lately it's been out of control. We have smart phones, smart TVs, smart cars, smart microwaves…but we have stupid people. All of the kids these days are out there with $700 cell phones, left to their own devices, thinking it is okay to perform tricks on camera just to see their videos 'go viral,' but none of them seem to have a lick of common sense or think these things through.

The other night, a teenager was brought in DOA. His parents were working at the time and trusted the young man to stay home alone, something that I also would have trusted of my own son at this young man's age. As many young teens do, this one invited over several friends as soon as his parents left. I stood by as law enforcement spoke to each of the three young men who had accompanied the ambulance. They admitted to watching lewd content on the television and smoking marijuana one of the teens found in his parents' bedroom.

Then the group moved to watching videos online of young people performing 'stunts.' Some of the stunts the young men detailed sounded downright dangerous, such as skateboarding off rooftops or young people daring one another to touch electricity lines with objects such as brooms or long branches.

The group viewed a video of 'fire breathers,' whom of which were trained professionals in the entertainment industry. The performers ingested a small amount of accelerant before holding a flame at their mouths. Then, the performer would spit the accelerant against the flame to create a fireball.

The young men in our ER waiting room showed law enforcement a video of the group acting out the same 'fire breathing' stunt. They had found lamp oil in the garage and used this as the accelerant. I will add my commentary momentarily on this piece of information alone. The young men then video-taped themselves spitting the lamp oil over a flame from a candle lighter, which then created large balls of fire that quickly extinguished. All of the young men commented following their turns that the accelerant left a 'taste' in their mouths.

Upon the patient's turn to perform the stunt, he was heard in the video as announcing he would be using more accelerant than used by his friends. I can only describe hearing this as understanding the patient wished to 'outdo' his friends, and he made a passing comment about posting the video on social media.

Judging from the video, I would estimate the patient held approximately four-to-six ounces of lamp oil in his mouth (as opposed to the swigs that the others used). He held up his lighter, with the flame inches from his lips, and the other gentlemen cheered him on.

In just one second, the patient made a face of disgust and it was apparent he had accidentally swallowed some of the lamp oil. He then coughed, which sent the remaining oil thrust forward in a forceful splatter. What went wrong here is that the patient was still experiencing the natural reflex of gagging and coughing, and in the moment the fireball was supposed to move forward, the patient gasped for air, which moved the flames down his windpipe and into his lungs. He was pronounced dead at the scene.

This is frightening on many levels, and for many reasons. For one, accelerant is not to be ingested. We often wonder why there are so many warning labels on common household products that any one of us would be intelligent enough not to do, but like you stated in your previous novel, someone had to have done it to get the warning label there. Accelerant can be absorbed and/or accidentally ingested. If this boy had not had passed away, he most likely would have vomited shortly after ingestion. Depending on if he would have swallowed more unintentionally, he very well may have ended up as a patient, anyway.

Secondly, the 'fire breathers' in the first video were professionally trained. I understand young minds do not often think things through, but I wish more people understood these acts performed by trained professionals should never be reenacted by untrained professionals. Fire breathing performers undergo years of training which includes what to do if something goes south. These young men simply thought something looked fun and thought they'd give it a try. As a result, one of their friends died a terrible death right in front of their eyes, and each one of those boys is still facing charges as an accomplice.

My message to everyone, even if I come off as sanctimonious or any other negative way to you or your readers is a this: parents, talk to your kids. Explain that even though it takes two seconds to send a nude picture, it can take years of counseling and numerous suicide attempts to live with the backlash. (I mention this because of the increase of such incidents.) Explain to your children that these 'viral videos' do not result in fame or fortune, but often others sharing them simply because they cannot believe how unfathomably dumb one person can be. Please explain that these stunts are incredibly dangerous and while we usually see positive outcomes, what we don't see are the videos when something goes terribly and shamefully wrong.

Please, if you use this, print that I am not attempting to bash the victim in this. I understand he was playing Monkey-See, Monkey-Do. But that game and the young group's attempts at going 'viral' took someone's life.

--N.A.
Texas

<u>Total Nightmare</u>

This isn't a funny story whatsoever, but I wanted to share with you my story to let you know you're not alone with holding up your emotions after a bad encounter.

I worked (yes, worked) as a medic for about five years at the time. We were called to a factory just on the edge of town. It's a small city, really. We don't have the big city luxuries like all-night food delivery or freeways, but the population is about 50,000, so it did take a few minutes to make it to the call.

We weren't in arms about the call on our way to it. The caller who'd contacted the 911 dispatcher said there was an accident involving boiling water, so we just thought we were dealing with another burn. The factory had a lot of minor complaints like that over time, and I'm pretty positive that was my third run out there in two days. We had a student riding along for a version of clinicals. He was hands-off, only there to watch. We couldn't just let him watch when we arrived on scene; my partner and I made him check on the bystanders who passed out or were vomiting or were sobbing so hard they couldn't breathe. I'm not sure it was our call to make, but my partner advised the unit's supervisor to evacuate the premises and he did.

This wasn't some minor burn to an arm or melted plastic splattering a cheek.

One of the employees had somehow gotten caught on a guardrail to an overhead balcony-type scaffold and had fallen 15-feet into a vat of boiling water. Even though it had taken us about six minutes to make the drive and probably about another minute or two to get in the building and to the scene, the man was still alive, even if just barely.

Someone had thought quickly and turned off the burner unit heating the vat, but nobody could get to the man because of the construction taking place around the open tub and its own construction. There was no way to get him out, other than standing on the same scaffolding from which he fell and using a pull-system my partner devised. It was made out of cinching straps collected from the rig and factory floor. Making the device probably took another five minutes, and trying to get the loop wrapped around the man's abdomen as he floated in the vat, whimpering, took a few minutes more. By the time my partner, the man's supervisor, our shadow, and I lifted the man from the vat, I thought he'd be dead, but as soon as we eased him to the scaffolding I realized he wasn't.

This man's skin had blistered and popped and burned. We tried to remove his clothing, but when we tried to take his safety gloves off, his skin degloved with them. We couldn't remove his work uniform without taking his skin, too.

He couldn't talk, and he couldn't move. I have no clue how he was still alive. For a few more minutes, we tried to get our stretcher up to the scaffolding but knew the only way to transport the man to the hospital was to somehow move him to the stretcher. We didn't know what to do. Thank God one of us was thinking straight at the time. The man shadowing us talked calmly to the man, calling him by name, and repeated to him that it was all going to be okay. You said in a few of your stories that you hate lying and wonder if the patients' families will ever know, and maybe it's different for the families, but I can tell you that sometimes it's a necessity in the field and all you can do for the patients themselves. In this case, it was all we could do, and I have to tell myself day in and day out that this patient appreciated the serenity our shadow was trying to offer. This isn't to say I don't question telling patients it's all going to be okay, but I always have to tell myself they deserve their final moments to be calm and as happy as we can make them, so if that means lying to someone and talking about family for the last five minutes of their lives, that has to mean something.

Our patient, not surprisingly, expired on scene. Overall, as you can imagine, it was a horrific ordeal and one that's become an inner demon. A few months after that call, I quit my job as a medic and transferred to dispatch. That was the worst thing I'd ever seen in my entire life, and I honestly don't know how people handle the ripples that come with situations like that. I can't even sit in a hot tub anymore and sometimes have panic attacks if the water in the shower is too hot.

The guy shadowing us went on to be an RN. He went on to work in a burn unit at a hospital upstate.

--R.K.

Wyoming

You Can't Make It Up

Quite a few readers submitted some *odd* stories about patients' reasons to call 911, visit the ER, or go to the doctor. Some are legitimate, others…wow. I've edited most down to tidbits, and well, here they are.

*

A family brought in their 80-something-year-old grandmother. The woman had been running a fever, experienced chills, and was vomiting frequently. She became a hassle until we listened to her and sent her family to the waiting room. The patient was experiencing an infection. She said she always wanted a nipple piercing and pierced her own nipple. It then became infected and her immune system could not fight the infection on its own. The patient had to spend two days in ICU, all for trying to wipe something from her bucket list.

--W.S.
California

*

A big, burly man made an appointment with my office for allergies. He came in wearing his biker gear and was covered in tattoos and piercings. If I saw him in a dark alley, I would have been afraid.

The man soon confessed that he didn't *really* have allergies. He just wanted me to write a note saying he did because his girlfriend wanted to adopt a cat and he didn't want her to know he was deathly afraid of them.

--N.W.
Utah

*

I'm a dental hygienist. Had a woman come in one time and tell me she couldn't get rid of her chronic halitosis and wanted me to check for bad teeth. She didn't have any. In fact, she had the nicest set of teeth I'd seen in a while, but man, she wasn't kidding about her bad breath. I had to keep turning my head and pretending to look at paperwork just to catch my breath.

I asked her what she used for her cleaning regiment. Ready?

A homemade paste made up of coconut oil, crushed garlic, vinegar, and baking soda. She used it multiple times, daily.

I advised her to switch to something that didn't contain garlic.

--K.M.
Idaho

*

I once had a mother rush in her young child and demand to be seen immediately because the child ingested a foreign object. She was literally pushing elderly patients out of the way and we had to move her to the side of lobby just to find out what was going on because she was becoming loud and even more aggressive, screaming the typical 'this is an emergency room and I shouldn't have to wait in line for an emergency' hoopla.

Her kid swallowed a loose tooth.

I guess that was *totally* worth knocking down a 92-year-old experiencing abdominal pain.

--D.E.
New Hampshire

*

No joke. I registered a patient once for a psych eval because he was 'distraught' over not having received an invitation letter from Hogwarts. He was probably 30, but he believed the Harry Potter books were real and he couldn't figure out why he didn't get his letter.

--S.P.
New York

\

*

All those cautionary urban legends are true. I went to a scene one time and had to move a dead man off of a prostitute. He had a heart attack and the woman under him couldn't roll out from under his 300-pound body. She screamed for help until someone in the next room of the motel called 911.

--M.R.R.
Florida

*

A single dad brought in his mortified 13-year-old daughter at two in the morning because she started her period and he didn't know what to do. One of our female nurses went in to explain to the girl all of the changes she was going to experience and how to use feminine products. Another nurse offered dad some coffee and tried to make him feel less embarrassed for not knowing how to handle the situation.

--L.K.

Iowa

*

A man came in for self-inflicted trauma and an emergency psych hold. He tried to cut off his tongue because he said it was a parasite that wasn't supposed to be in his body.

--B.D.

Kentucky

*

I had an underage patient one night who lied about her age and name at the registration desk to be seen without a parent. I recognized her right away from seeing her in the paper for winning an award at her high school. She was crying and wanted to know if there was any kind of medicine I could give her to make her breasts grow in size because none of the boys at school were interested in her 'flat chest.' I had to send her home because I couldn't treat that type of complaint for a minor and felt horrible that she was so upset.

--F.K.M.

Vermont

*

I work in a small clinic and we used to hand patients a form to fill out, which included a line for the patients to write-in his/her own chief complaint(s).

'Snack bit.'

It took three receptionists and an NP ten minutes to figure out the patient meant he'd been bitten by a snake.

We stopped using those forms because we could hardly ever figure out why patients were there, unless we tracked them down and asked them.

--B.B.

Mississippi

*

Had a guy come in and tell me he was part of Al Qaeda and listed Lindsay Lohan as his emergency contact, but he couldn't list her phone number because she dropped her phone in the Mediterranean Sea during the last cruise they took…Yeah.

--P.A.
California

*

So, I once had this guy who learned the hard way not to use Icy Hot to masturbate.

--B.P.
Ohio

*

During my first day on surgery, this woman was sent to the Unit Clerk's area to ask what she needed to do for us to close up her belly button. I didn't know what to say so I told her to go to the ER, but she said they sent her up to me. Nothing was wrong with her navel. She just didn't want to have a belly button anymore. I told her to talk to her primary doctor and start from there.

--S.R.

Washington, D.C. vicinity

Problem Child

I work for Child Services and was on call to respond to a child abduction and abuse case. When I arrived at the hospital, I was briefed on the case, involving an eight-year-old. A man involved was in a trauma room, badly beaten. The child was placed in a separate holding area. It was my job to interview both.

Several police officers were in the room with the adult, so I went to the holding room to speak to the child, who was happily eating a popsicle and watching cartoons.

The girl told me her mother allowed her to walk to a nearby grocery store to purchase candy with money she had received for her upcoming birthday. She was approached by a 'bad man' who tried to 'take' her. She said she learned in school to scream things like "Stranger!" and "Help!" so that other 'good' adults would recognize there was a problem and step in to offer assistance.

I informed the child this was the right thing for her to have done in the situation, but I noted she did not seem a bit afraid, so I wanted to touch down on that. I told her I would have been afraid if that happened to me. She told me she wasn't afraid. I then told her I would be afraid if my mommy wasn't there with me. Again, she told me she wasn't afraid.

I stepped out of the room to inquire about the nurses contacting the girl's mother. They were unable to do so because the child could not remember her phone number or her address, so I was informed that some of the police officers were looking into contacting the child's mother.

When I went back in the holding room, something just didn't feel right, so I sat down again and asked the child to tell me her story once more. She didn't miss a single word from the first time she told it. She maintained she was at the grocery store to purchase candy, when a 'bad man' tried to take her. She screamed for help and screamed that the man was a stranger.

Then the child began telling me about how 'good men' from the grocery store stopped the 'bad man' from taking her. She recollected aloud how the 'good men' pushed and hit the 'bad man' and then the police showed up to help more.

Again, I left the room to see where we stood on finding the child's mother and I wanted to speak to the man in the trauma room. Something wasn't settling well with me regarding this case.

I was allowed to enter the man's room and was quickly informed by him that the child *was* his daughter and she had thrown a tantrum because he wouldn't buy her what she wanted. When he tried to leave the store with her, she began shouting out for help, which prompted other shoppers and grocery baggers to assault him and remove the child from the scene. He was arrested on attempted kidnapping, even though he told the arresting officers the same story he told me, all because the girl in the holding room repeated her story with such accuracy and denied she knew the man.

The man had given the police officers his wife's work phone number, and she soon arrived to the hospital. It was a mess, though, still, because there were suspicions that the child was not actually their child. The little girl said the woman was not her mother and acted afraid of her.

The child's mother voluntarily offered DNA and offered to go home to get the child's birth certificate from the family's file cabinet. She returned with not only a birth certificate, but also with family photos from the time the child was a baby.

It took an hour after mom submitted a cheek swab for the child to break down and admit she threw a tantrum in the store to 'get [her] dad in trouble' and she saw on TV that if you say you're kidnapped you can get whatever you want, so she lied and did get what she wanted.

The girl's parents explained the child had been visiting a child therapist in attempts to get her behavioral problems properly diagnosed.

That was the strangest, most frustrating case I've ever had. I am the most dedicated child rights advocate you'll ever meet, but I really wanted to spank that girl before I left. The bad part of all of it is that I think there was something so deeply seeded in her mind that I'm not sure that she even cared what kind of mess she caused for her parents or the police department.

--N.K.
Illinois

Let's Take a Break

ER vet of 37 years here, and the funniest story I had probably won't be funny to a lot of other people, but I'm giving it a shot.

Two college girls came in years ago, with one complaining of nausea and pelvic cramping. Charge assigned the patient to me, and I went in to ask the routine questions. I was exhausted and wanted to get right down to it, so I worked on the assumption that the patient was experiencing menstrual discomfort or was pregnant.

I asked the patient when her last period was, and she told me it was late, but she should be on it now.

Check mark on the 'you're probably pregnant' paper, yes?

"Are you sexually active?" I asked.

The patient nodded. Her friend sat in a chair and just listened patiently.

Another check mark.

"And are you using birth control pills or any other form of contraceptives?"

The patient shook her head.

Check three.

"So I'm going to go get a pregnancy test and have you go in the restroom down the hall," I told her.

"But I'm not pregnant," the girl said. "I can't be."

I tried not to yawn as I explained to this young woman that if you: 1.) are sexually active, 2.) do not use birth control, 3.) your menstrual cycle is late, and 4.) you come to the ER at midnight because you're experiencing cramping and nausea, yes, you can become pregnant and the signs were pointing in that direction.

The patient's friend started to giggle and I shot her a confused, angry look.

"I can't be pregnant because this is my girlfriend," the patient told me. "She's the one I have sex with. So I can't be pregnant."

I was so embarrassed with my behavior that I excused myself and went to talk to the doctor. He told me to administer a pregnancy test, anyway, just so they could rule it out as a factor, and when it came back negative he'd come in the room. He said this as he was eating fried chicken, so in hindsight I'm sure he just wanted to buy himself a few minutes to finish his supper.

When I went back to the room with a pregnancy test, the patient was irate. She threw a pillow at me and called me several bad names. Finally, I laid down the law and told her to continue the exam, we'd have to rule out pregnancy. She snatched the test from my hands and went to the restroom while her girlfriend and I waited for her return.

The patient's girlfriend was incredibly pleasant to speak to, and I wish I would have had her as a patient instead. Then I started thinking that if she were the patient the actual patient would probably have been the nice one, just because there's like some unwritten rule of nursing that says if one person in the room is nice to you, it's never going to be the patient.

Anyway, the patient was taking a while to return, so I excused myself from the conversation I was having with her girlfriend and walked to the restroom. I could hear the patient sobbing loudly, so I knocked on the door. She opened it and showed me the test.

"Two lines means I'm pregnant, right?" she cried.

I nodded.

She freaked out and declared the test was wrong and that she came to the wrong hospital to help her. I assured the patient we were all there to help, but she still wanted to leave. I went back to her room after she dressed and had her sign her discharge papers.

She let it slip that she was pregnant and the pleasant girlfriend wasn't so pleasant anymore. The two started arguing in the room and took it to the hall. Someone paged our janitor (we didn't have security back then) and he tried to explain to the women that fighting would not be tolerated in the facility, so the patient's girlfriend just said, "Fine," and left the patient at the hospital.

This was back before we had cell phones, so we had to track down phone books for the dorms and when the patient couldn't reach anyone to pick her up, she called her mother collect and had to wait three hours for her mother to take her back home.

I really don't have a clue what happened to these women or the baby.

--C.G.

Michigan

<u>Reminders from Emergency Service Providers</u>

Alongside the funny, sad, and scary submissions came tips, venting, secret confessions, and hints from frustrated nurses, doctors, police officers, and medics. Keep in mind that almost every point/bullet is from a different reader.

- If I ask you if you're on meds and you say no, don't tell me five minutes later, "But I do take Clonazepam three times a week." That means you *are* on meds.

- When I ask if you're taking medication, I mean *your* medication, prescribed to *you*. If your buddy slips you pills on the low, though, go ahead and tell me about it so I don't kill you by mixing in a different medication.

- Why are you cussing me out for not doing anything for your mother, but you're the one who waited four days to bring her in when you thought she was having a stroke? There's only so much we can do, and yes, some of it could have been done if you brought your family member in right when the symptoms began.

- Most people try to talk me out of ticketing them for traffic violations, and that's to be expected. What I can't stand is when drivers become angry or violent when I'm writing a speeding ticket. My first-ever call was responding to an accident caused when a speeding driver went off the road and rolled his minivan. Not only was he killed, but so was his four-month-old son. Someone had to notify the driver's wife that her husband and baby died. So maybe, just maybe, when an officer is ticketing you or even giving you a warning, keep in mind that maybe he or she is trying to save your life by preventing something he or she couldn't prevent before.

- Let me tell you something: if you came in for real pain but it's not that bad at the moment, don't ask for pain meds. What's going to happen is I'm going to give you all I can, it's going to start to wear off (but not enough to give you more), and then you're going to writhe in pain until the doctor gives the okay to give you more (if that even happens). My suggestion (which is not a medical suggestion but personal) is to wait until your pain is about a four or five. Any less, the meds will make you high and you'll have to wait out the time until you can get more meds. Any higher, the meds aren't going to be as effective for you.

- I get patients who treat me like I went to medical school and failed out before I could become a doctor. That's not what happened with 99.9-percent of nurses in the field. Please show us a little respect. We wanted to become nurses to help people, not get insulted on a daily basis.

- One thing I've learned in all my years is to pay attention to the patient who doesn't bother you or complain or ask for anything. This is usually the patient who needs your attention the most, but he or she is too afraid of 'bugging' you. About 85-percent of the chemo patients I see won't ask for pain meds because they don't want to be a bother, but I've had men with hangnails walk in and ask for morphine while I was doing chest compressions.

- As a physician, I do my best to never yell or correct a nurse in front of other staff members or patients, and I won't tolerate anyone else doing it either. My mother was a nurse and came home in tears one afternoon because the doctor yelled at her in front of everyone and her patients stopped trusting her. It ruined her entire month and the older I became, I noticed it seemed to ruin a part of her, too.

- I am a nursing supervisor and I wish I could tell staff (and patients) this: If you go out to eat and your order is incorrect, you first try to speak with the store manager before complaining to corporate, correct? I want to help everyone and I do try my best, but if you can handle your complaints by speaking to the floor Charge, do that instead of calling me because a patient's family wants to complain that the cafeteria is closed.

- Some people reviewing your books seem angry that you don't give follow-ups regarding your patients, but I work in Pediatrics and can confirm we rarely hear from patients again. I wish parents would update us more often or bring the kids in for a visit every now and then. We really miss our patients when they're gone and wonder how they're getting along once they're feeling better.

- Sometimes we think you're going to die, but we're not going to tell you that because the human spirit is essential to healing progression.

- If you're truly in pain and we don't recognize your requests for pain meds (if you can have any), ask for someone else. A nurse on my floor was fired because she withheld pain meds and was caught telling patients their pain 'wasn't that bad' and to 'suck it up.'

- Don't feel stupid if you don't understand what we're telling you. Yes, we do tease with each other at the station to pass time, but our very first concern is making sure our patients are taken care of. We can break it down so that you can understand it. We need you to be honest if there's something you can't understand on your discharge papers because if you are confused about something that means your condition can become even worse and quickly. By the way, we have to look up stuff, too, so don't feel like you can't ask us questions.

- I don't know how you don't know that you smell so bad. Then I wonder if you do. If you're having trouble making ends meet for hygiene products or need a place to shower, tell me or tell the doctor or tell the CNA. A lot of hospitals have showers and deodorants, soaps, and other toiletries for patients to use. The worst anyone can do is tell you no. But if you don't even try, you're going to keep getting sick, and I can guarantee that.

- If a patient tells me he drinks two drinks per weekend, I mentally double that because nobody ever tells the truth about addiction unless they're at rock bottom. I trust a homeless drunk's honesty about his addiction more than I can trust a business man's.

- I hear 'I can't' a lot. You *can't* quit smoking before a spot shows up on your lung scan, and then you *can't* quit smoking when it does. You *can't* quit drinking three-2 liters of soda a day before you become diabetic, and then you *can't* quit when you're faced with diabetic complications. You *can't* quit drinking alcohol before you get a DUI, and then you *can't* quit when you lost your license. It's simple: you *can* quit, you just *won't*. I've quit all three and can tell you it *can* be done. You just have to *want* it. Stop giving everyone excuses. You have to decide if the things that make you happy in your life are worth quitting for. Don't be afraid to find a sponsor, even if it's not alcohol you're trying to quit. Just stop coming up with excuses because all I'm starting to hear is, "It's okay if I die."

- If I'm not at the hospital, I'm not your nurse. If you see me wearing street clothes in the hospital, I'm not your nurse. And what's up with these BS mandatory meetings on my only day off, that always seem to fall during the time I'd be asleep and last about 20 minutes?

- I will do my best to explain your family member's condition, but when I receive calls from 20 of your family members, it prevents me from caring for your ill relative. It makes me wonder how well you all get along because everyone seems to know at least one key point of care, but nobody in the group fully knows what's going on. Sometimes I want to tell you to call each other and then when you need more information to call me. I can't do that.

- Unspoken way of the ER: if the patient requires isolation and you must wear/take off PPE gear each time you interact with said patient, he or she will ring the call bell more than all your other patients combined. You might as well just put one person on standby with the sole purpose of gearing up and answering the bell so coworkers can deal with the other patients.

- After ten years in emergency services, I'm starting to think we should keep free pregnancy tests in the waiting room. I bet that would cut down on our times.

- Sometimes I want to throw a handful of pills at the seekers and tell them to leave, just so I don't have to listen to another fabricated sob story about how Jennifer's ex-mother-in-law's husband came over and tripped over the baby's rattle and knocked over the pill bottle and 36 Oxys fell down the drain.

- Many times over the years I have been on the receiving end of hearing from patients that my professional diagnoses are incorrect, simply because the patients and/or families 'Googled' possibly causations of present symptoms. Some even have gone as far to inform me the treatment plans I have developed were incorrect, also based on 'Googling' treatments. Perhaps seven years of medical school and nearly $200,000 of debt was a waste of time.

- "Well, if I gave her Tylenol you wouldn't know that her fever was this high." Hmmm. If you gave her Tylenol, maybe her fever would had gone away and you wouldn't need to be in the emergency room at two in the morning.

- If I ask, "What seems to be the problem today, Mrs. X?" and you bitterly snap something of the sorts, "If I knew I wouldn't need you," please be aware that you just added five minutes to each of your requests during your time on my watch. Poor manners due to fear or pain, I can excuse, but I won't tolerate anyone's general saltiness.

- I'm sick of people treating the ER like a free pantry of food and supplies. It's one thing if you're in need, but the next college kid I get who comes in asking for free chap stick and lotion and wants to take home three boxes of tissues and rolls of toilet paper from our bathroom just because he doesn't want to buy the things like everyone else in the world, I might just snap and slap him. If you need help, tell us. If you'd rather take from us so you can use your money for booze and movies, take the begging someplace else.

<u>You Should Know</u>

We had this meds-seeker we were all familiar with. He'd come in sometimes three or four times a day, and he knew us all by name. This man paid attention to shift changes, and when he couldn't get high during one shift, he'd go home and wait until the next shift. His excursions were not exclusive to our facility; he was well known by the staff located around the city's other hospitals and clinics.

His drug of choice was Dilaudid. Headache? Dilaudid. Rectal pain? Dilaudid. Stubbed toe? Dilaudid. You get the picture. He often resorted to self-inflicting injuries to receive a shot or prescription for the drug.

After (yet another) failed attempt to obtain a high, the man left the ER, visibly angrier than usual. He punched a wall on the way out. I reckoned he was going through withdrawals, so I called the nearest hospital and gave the receptionist a warning.

About fifteen minutes after our guy left, I got a call from Walgreens.

"I need to verify a prescription," the woman said.

"The doctor is busy right now, but if you give me the info I can find him and call you back."

"No, I'll wait."

I rolled my eyes. "Okay, what's it for?"

She laughed a little. "Uh, I think it's for Dilaudid."

"You think?"

"Well, it's spelled d-i-e-l-a-w-d-i-e-d. I couldn't help but think that Dr. X knew how to spell that, but I thought I'd check."

I laughed.

Our meds-seeker swiped a prescription pad on his way out and when he was arrested he had already written six prescriptions for himself.

-S.T.

Idaho

<u>Ow, Ow, Ow</u>

We were called to an apartment complex for a 20-year-old male with penile bleeding. Nobody would tell us what happened. Dispatch kept laughing when we'd ask, so we dropped it and went to the scene.

Inside the apartment, we found a young woman wrapped in bedsheets, sitting on the floor outside the bathroom. She was crying and there was blood around her mouth and dried in big drips down her chest. We asked her what happened, but she was crying too hard to tell us.

I could hear a guy inside the bathroom groaning and occasionally screaming out in pain, so I tried to go in, but the door was locked.

I identified myself and tried to get the guy to open the bathroom door, but he kept telling me it was too embarrassing, in between telling me he was 'going to lose [his penis]'.

"Someone tell me what's going on," I shouted, out of patience.

Losing my temper didn't help the situation any. The girl on the floor got scared and went to the bedroom, where she continued crying. The guy in the bathroom yelled at me for yelling.

"I can't help you if I can't see you," I said to him through the closed door.

I heard the door lock click, so I opened the door. There was blood all over the place-on the floor, in the tub, smeared on the sink...it looked like someone had been butchered in there.

That wasn't the shocking part.

This guy was holding his penis with both hands as blood squirted out all over. His hands were slippery from the blood and he was losing color in his face.

"What happened?" I exclaimed.

He then passed out and hit his head on the toilet.

I yelled for my partner and we transported the guy to the ER with lights and sirens. My partner was a male and seemed uneasy with the patient, so he drove and I stayed in the back of the rig.

"What happened?" asked the nurse who took the patient.

I shrugged and explained nobody would tell us. She used smelling salts to bring him back to consciousness after he repeatedly passed out.

Finally, we could get the whole story.

The man picked up a cute girl at the bar and took her back to his place for sex. She began performing fellatio on the man.

Here's how it went terribly wrong: the female had braces, and the man had the 'Jacob's Ladder' piercings. If you don't know what this is, it's a series of barbell piercings that run up the shaft of the penis. I think the man had four or five barbells inserted in his penis before fellatio. The woman's braces caught on two of the barbells, and when they both panicked, two of the piercings were torn straight out.

The patient had to undergo a lengthy surgery to repair the shaft of his penis. I bet he'll be more careful in the future.

--E.K.

Florida

My not-so-favorite patients are the ones who are found unconscious in the streets, yards, or outside of bars, piss-drunk, and when they wake up in the ED they get angry and say, "I didn't ask for anyone to bring me here, so I'm not paying."

Well, usually you have to be *able* to refuse transport, but next time you want to get slammed and die on the side of Hooters with a BAC five times the legal limit, I'll try to remember that.

--D.A.

Nevada

I Ain't Afraid of No Goat...Maybe

We saw on a chart from day shift a chief complaint of, "Bitten by goat, involved in MVA."

Was the patient bitten by a goat, who was riding as a passenger in his vehicle, and therefore wrecked?

Was the patient bitten by a goat, and during his getaway he wrecked?

Was the comma trying to tell us the goat was involved in the MVA?

We were curious and I can confirm the betting pool thing you talk about is a real occurrence because we were collecting bets from the nurse's lounge as to what happened with the patient. We were so eager to know that one of our people called the day shift nurse and asked.

The patient had been working on a farm for the first time, trying to secure extra funds for when he returned to college after summer ended. He entered a pen containing milk goats and moved in too close to baby goats, so the mother attacked him. When the mother attacked, other goats from the opposite side of the pen also attacked. During the attempt to fight them off, he was bitten multiple times by (what he believed to be) the mother goat. He was not entirely positive of which goat bit him because he was scared and trying to get away.

Hearing the patient making so much commotion, the farmer's wife emerged from an adjacent barn and shooed the goats away, thus allowing the patient to escape. Seeing that several of the bites had ripped chunks of flesh from the farmhand's forearms, the farmer's wife instructed the man to ride as a passenger to the ER. The farm would be responsible for any bills, and they offered the man cash compensation to avoid a lawsuit. The man agreed to this.

On the way to the hospital, the farmer's wife swerved to miss a stray dog in the center of her lane. She overcorrected her steering and the car rolled off the side of the road and down a hill.

The nurse also told us that 'if we had looked instead of calling her at home,' we'd all had seen the patient was admitted to the CCU for a punctured lung, in addition to his bites, which some needed grafting to heal.

We didn't ask about the farmer's wife because the nurse was already mad that we called her at home.

--O.B.
North Dakota

<u>Denial</u>

A man came in with his mother because he had a chief complaint of chest pain. We knew he'd had a history of substance abuse (i.e. cocaine) because we'd dealt with his ODs, withdrawals, and jail clearances over time.

"John, have you been using cocaine again?" the doctor asked.

"Not for a year now."

"We're going to run a blood-tox just to rule out substance abuse and check your levels, okay?"

The patient agreed to this.

It wasn't a big surprise when the tox screen came back detailing high levels of cocaine.

"John," the doctor said, "I thought you told me you haven't used cocaine in a year?"

The patient popped his eyes open and said, "I haven't."

"Well, your results came back with high traces of cocaine."

At this point, the patient's mother started scolding him and lecturing that she was only paying half of his rent and trying to help him get back on his feet because he swore he wasn't abusing drugs again.

"My friends do it when they come over," he said. "It must have absorbed through my skin when I was sitting on the couch telling them drugs aren't the way."

The doctor laughed, shook his head, and started to speak, but he walked out when the patient's mother hugged him and said, "Oh, I knew you weren't doing drugs again."

--P.K.

New Jersey

And an EMS/ER Bill

I'm a nurse and one time I opened my cell phone bill and passed out—hit my head on the kitchen counter and everything. Thankfully, my 12-year-old knew to call 911 and I was still unconscious when EMS arrived.

I passed out because the same 12-year-old who'd called 911 went on some app on her brand-new cell phone and somehow charged up $12,000 to my credit card by purchasing in-game money and in-game extras.

I'm caught in between laughing more at the stories people tell me or trying not to laugh because I know how it is.

By the way, I disputed the charges but my cell company only agreed to remove half of the charges, so I was still stuck with a $6,000 phone bill.

Wild Goose Chase

I work on the Psychiatric unit and we took a guy from the ER. He was exhibiting violent tendencies, and despite him being in his late-70s, he was rather strong and had to be restrained to protect staff.

He was hollering that he was cold, so I went to take him an extra blanket.

No crap, this guy looked over to me and said, "Miss, please call law enforcement. I would like to confess now."

I was just an intern at the time, so I asked, "Confess to what?"

"Murder," he told me.

I freaked out and left to get someone in charge. The man repeated to my superior that he wanted to confess to murdering several women. My superior called the cops, and when they arrived the man detailed gruesome murders that took place between the 1970s and into the 80s. Then he started giving locations of where he dumped the bodies.

Soon we had FBI agents on our ward. It was a big to-do at the hospital because we aren't located in some huge city. We're actually kind of between the middle of nowhere and hours away from a major airport. So, it was crazy to have FBI agents asking for coffee refills or how to get to the cafeteria.

Well, the FBI sent out a team of excavators to find the bodies the patient confessed to killing. This man knew patient names, where they were abducted, their ages, appearances, and everything about the cases. But no bodies were showing up, which left the FBI confused and frustrated. They gave the man a polygraph in his room and he passed it.

The only problem with all of this was the man never actually killed anyone. The FBI called in their own counselor and determined the man was mentally ill and was delusional. He was young when the murders took place and the counselor said he seemed to have an eerie obsession with the murders, but there was no reason to believe he killed the women.

Someone was able to reach the patient's family after an extended period of time and it turned out that the patient's son stopped talking to him because all the patient talked about were serial killers. The man's son brought in a tote filled with scrapbooks the man had kept. In each scrapbook were newspaper clippings with articles about serial killers. The patient started confessing to all the murders, which would make him at least three different serial killers, even one whom which was captured and executed.

The patient was released to a supervised nursing home.

--K.R.
Illinois

Heartbreaking

I have been a NICU nurse for one year, and I have already experienced my fill of bad parents. Now, some parents are wonderful. They are joys to be around and seem to shower their precious babies with love and prayers. Some parents yell at you because you try to explain that the baby is not stable enough to come out of the incubator or the immune system could be compromised. Others bring ill family members up on the floor and we can't tell they're ill until they're already around the babies. I thought things like that were enough to tick me off when I first started.

A few months ago, a baby was brought to our unit after being born at 22-weeks of gestation. This is a miracle in itself, that the baby was alive and appeared to be striving to thrive. The baby was just under one-pound. We couldn't even find diapers in our supply closet to fit this baby, so someone from the OB floor brought in doll diapers from her daughter's old dolls. Even these were too large for the baby, but we fooled around with them until they fit decently.

During the first few days of the baby's admission to my floor, two or three people came up to the unit clerk's desk to see the child, but they refused to put on isolation gear, so we turned them away. By the end of the week, nobody showed up to visit the child. We asked about the baby's mother and were told she was having a difficult time recovering from her preterm labor. This is something we understood. One of the OB nurses gave us the mother's cell phone number and we sent her daily pictures and updates via text.

One of the nurses called the baby's mother and the mom said she couldn't get to the NICU to see her baby because she lived four hours away and only delivered at our hospital because she was passing through our city. She said she had no way to get back to visit her baby. So, being nice, the nurse volunteered to drive to the mother's house, bring her to the NICU, and even pay for two weeks of a motel rental. Others on our floor heard of the kind gesture and chipped in to pay for mom's food and to extend the motel rental.

The mother declined.

After a few weeks of going back and forth with the mother, we learned she 'didn't want' the baby. CPS became involved. The mother said she didn't want a sick child and she didn't want to have all the bills to pay for a kid that came from an unplanned pregnancy. It broke my heart. The only love this child knew came from dedicated, around-the-clock nurses.

A husband and husband came last week to see their new child in person. They just signed the adoption papers and have already been to see the baby five times. The baby still has a long way before discharge and the doctor said the baby will probably have to wear glasses and may have complications with immunity, but otherwise should be a 'normal' child.

I pray each night this never happens again because I don't know if I'm cut out for this line of nursing. I can't understand how anyone could just 'not want' their own child anymore.

-S.C.

Mississippi

Embarrassing

I can definitely relate to your story about the nurse and the amputee. Here's what I did. I'm a registration clerk, too, by the way.

Patient says to me while I'm on the phone with Life Line: "I think I need some help. I lost a few of my pigs from the market."

Me, mindlessly responding as I was trying to listen to the ETA of the helicopter and thinking the patient needed mental health: "Okay, just have a seat for me and we'll get you a counselor to talk to in just a second."

Patient, confused: "I don't need a counselor. I lost some of my fingers."

Me, still not offering my full attention: "Well, where did you last see them?"

Patient, now angry, holds up a hand wrapped in a bloody towel and says: "Chopped off by a saw. Now, can I get some help?"

I was so embarrassed by not paying attention to the patient and apologized until I was blue in the face. He took it well but reminded me that he wasn't paying enough attention when he accidentally cut three of his fingers off, either.

--C.C.
Ohio

Out of This World

I transferred to OB from Pediatrics and my very first patient down there was the oddest I've seen in my entire career.

So, this woman was brought up from the ER registration area. She was in active labor, overdue at 41 weeks. And she was crazy.

I mean that. She had several mental illnesses professionally diagnosed and had been off her anti-psychotic medication since her second trimester, so by the time she made it to Labor and Delivery to have the baby, she was so far beyond the deep end that she was probably in the ocean.

To make matters a lot worse, the patient's boyfriend recently broke up with her and she didn't have nearby family, so while we waited for her mother to make the drive to the hospital, we had to work diligently to try to calm the patient. She didn't want to sleep, and she refused pain medication. Setting up her IV for fluids was a nightmare.

The patient was completely convinced that the child she was carrying was an alien hybrid. She told everyone she saw that she was abducted during her first trimester and aliens took her 'real' baby and replaced it with a baby from a test tube. She said that baby was a product of alien testing, where the aliens took healthy fetuses from pregnant women, injected them with DNA, kept the fetuses in test tubes until they could prove viable, and then the aliens would abduct another pregnant woman, take her fetus, and place a hybrid in her womb.

We tried to reason with the woman that she showed no signs of surgery and we did a bedside ultrasound to ease her mind, but even though the ultrasound showed a healthy (human) baby, the woman screamed and told us to turn off the monitor. All she could see was an alien baby.

When the patient's mother arrived, we learned she had temporary medical power of attorney over the patient, so she asked that for the safety of the patient and the baby that we sedated the patient. We gave her a quick shot to help her sleep. She ended up having vaginal birthing complications, so we conducted a caesarean.

The patient returned about three months later with her perfectly healthy human child and apologized to us. She said she couldn't remember everything she said but from what she could remember, it embarrassed her. She started taking her medications after choosing to bottle feed and no longer believed her daughter was an alien hybrid.

--B.A.
Wisconsin

I had to run in on my day off because I left my book there and needed it to study. As I was leaving, I saw on the board a chief complaint of "Penis stuck in condiment bottle."

I still don't know what that was about because I just didn't care at that point, but I wonder every day of my life what the hell people are doing with their lives and how they make these decisions that end up as stories in books like yours.

--P.M.E.
Utah

I work surgery admissions and it's part of my job to ask, "And you've been fasting, correct?" or something like that to verify patients haven't eaten prior to surgery.

One guy told me he had performed oral sex on his girlfriend and wanted me to check with the nurse to make sure he could still have his surgery.

He was dead-serious.

--L.W.

Washington

Three in the morning, during the middle of a snowstorm—when 10 MVAs have come in within 30 minutes—is *obviously* the best time to come to the ER because you're concerned that you've been going bald for two years.

--D.N.

Kansas

You Don't Eat it, Silly

I work in a small city and we get all the people you talk about in your books and then some, but my most memorable case from recent was this mom who brought in her little boy. The mom noticed her kids were too quiet and went to check on them. She found her oldest son (5) spraying Silly String in her youngest son's mouth. She screamed for the two to stop and told the youngest to spit out the product, but he was two and I know you said you don't have kids, but if you've been around them you know they don't always listen so well.

Mom took the can from her oldest and realized it was about half empty. There was no string around the room, so when she asked where it went, her oldest son laughed and pointed to the string-eater.

We called Poison Control and they verified the product did contain toxic chemicals that should not be ingested. By the time we could get to the part of the call where the hotline operator recommended treatment, the two-year-old was vomiting uncontrollably. It was horrible to watch because he was crying and you could tell this poor boy had no idea what to do or why this was happening. His mom was sobbing and panicking, screaming pleas for us not to let her baby die. The doctors we had that night consulted one another and agreed that the best course of action was to not give the baby medication to stop the vomiting because he needed to purge the string and chemicals from his system.

What we didn't think about was the fact that the chemicals coming out had to travel through the child's body, mainly his esophagus. After about thirty minutes of constant vomiting, the boy began spitting up blood with the vomit, and his mother lost it. We had to remove her from the room because she was a mess and was interfering with our attempts to keep the baby as calm as possible. We wanted her to be by his side, but she was refusing to let us place an IV for fluids—not due to religion preferences or such—but because she thought that meant her son was dying.

We called an on-call doc from Peds and he came in to help. He was quick to determine that the boy's bleeding stemmed from the chemicals in the Silly String irritating the boy's throat. The chemicals were basically burning this child's esophagus each time he vomited. We gave him milk to help coat his throat—do not allow your child or anyone who has ingested toxic chemicals to ingest anything and do not induce vomiting until you have consulted with Poison Control or a physician.

After an hour and a half of vomiting nonstop, the boy seemed to have the product out of his stomach and he fell asleep. We pushed fluids like no tomorrow because he was dehydrated from the vomiting. He did wake up and ask for a drink, but we had to hold off on that because we weren't sure if his stomach had truly settled, and we didn't want to cause him even more grief. He was transferred to our Pediatric ICU wing and was under observation for two days before he was discharged.

This is not a warning against the Silly String product whatsoever. It's just a reminder that even the most 'harmless,' fun products can do some serious damage if used incorrectly.

--S.F.

Arkansas

A 30-something-year-old man came in one night because he ran his tongue over his teeth and some of them felt pointy when he thought they were supposed to be flat. He wanted us to examine his mouth and make sure his teeth weren't growing into fangs.

I didn't order a psych consult because he wasn't mentally disturbed, just stupid.

--P.A., M.D.
South Dakota

<u>Uh, Ew</u>

My next patient had a complaint of 'thinks she's pregnant.' I think she was only the fourteenth patient to come in that night to want a pregnancy test.

Kerry, this girl didn't want a pregnancy test. She didn't even think she was pregnant.

The patient told me she wanted to have sex with her boyfriend but they were out of condoms, so they had unprotected sex. She wasn't on birth control and was afraid of becoming pregnant.

She asked me if I could 'scrape the stuff' out of her.

After a good two minutes of looking at her like she was dumb, I left the room and came back with a prescription for Plan-B.

--P.I.

Missouri

Uh, Double-Ew

When I in the end-run of my residency, I was questioning a middle-age woman about her pelvic and abdominal pain.

Her pain history started roughly four months prior to her ED visit. She rated the pain a 7/10. She complained of vaginal itching, burning, and discharge.

At this point, I was thinking the patient had contracted an STD or UTI.

"Are you sexually active?" I asked.

She shook her head.

"Were you sexually active when this pain began?" I asked.

She offered a sheepish expression. I had to coax her to speak to me honestly, giving the spiel about how there's nothing to be embarrassed about and there's nothing we haven't seen in the ED.

The patient then confessed she regularly inserted foreign objects in her vagina to receive pleasure because she could not afford sex toys. When I asked her to elaborate, under the impression that perhaps now we were looking at a case of pierced uterine lining, she listed items such as hairbrush handles, a (cool) curling iron, taper candles, and…a whisk.

I did my best not to come off as judgmental, though all I could think of was how I was going to start my story to the M.D. I was following.

I excused myself from the room and told the ED doctors what the woman had told me. They looked confused but shook it off and ordered pelvic and abdominal x-rays. When the tech brought the films to us, she was giggling so hard she was crying. I knew it had to be good because she was usually collected and not much got to her.

The x-rays showed a small whisk…yes, whisk, the kitchen utensil…lodged in the patient's vaginal cavity. The patient's mucosa had essentially 'swallowed' pieces of the utensil in the body's natural attempt to either absorb or discharge a foreign body. In this case, I can only assume the patient's body could not discharge the whisk and therefore attempted to absorb it.

We sent the patient to emergency surgery to remove the utensil, after she admitted to 'losing' it inside of herself months earlier and 'forgetting' it was there.

--P.L., M.D.
South Carolina

The scariest thing I've seen in my career on Psych was a patient who'd crushed a plastic cup to cut himself and was caught masturbating, using his blood as lubricant.

--B.W.

Arizona

We had to call expiration on a hit and run patient and no more than a minute later, a woman came to the curtain from the next room and asked if the man was an organ donor and wondered, since he'd passed away and her husband needed a kidney, if we could bypass the waiting list if the deceased patient was a match.

I was so mad that I had to leave the building.

--Name and location withheld at request

Number of submissions I have received regarding the chief complaint of 'small penis' or 'penis appears smaller than it used to be': 11.

ELEVEN!

That's a Way to Learn

(Author's note: This is the only story I've received from a member of the fire department.)

We were closer to the river than any other responders, so we took a truck out to the center of the bridge to respond to a call of a jumper. Callers stated a male in his early-to-mid-20s was seen leaping from a bridge located on the way out of town. I thought it was going to end in calling a team to fish his body out of the waters because all week it had been about 30-degrees and the river was full of large boulders and logs.

When we arrived on scene, the man was flopping around in the river's center, screaming for help. I was honestly shocked that the 15-foot leap to the river didn't injure him severely or fatally, but there he was, every few moments swept away by the current and occasionally yanked under the water, only to swim awkwardly back to his starting point, where he continued to scream.

We were able to get a team down the side of the bridge and to the western bank. It didn't occur to us until we were on the bank that we had a truck supply check earlier and someone had forgotten to place some of our water-rescue supplies back on the rack, so we were working with one rope bag that contained 30-feet of rope, our fire gear, and gloves. I didn't know how we were going to get the jumper out of the river because 30-feet of rope wasn't going to reach him, and when we yelled at him to try to swim closer, he screamed back that he didn't know how to swim, so he couldn't do anything but stay in the spot he was in.

Yes, ma'am. This man planned to commit suicide by jumping off a bridge, and when the leap didn't kill him, his natural urge to preserve his life kicked in and he surprisingly learned to keep himself afloat and how to swim just enough to keep him in a safe spot, until someone could rescue him.

One of the guys with me started to wade in the waters, but when the water reached his knees he knew it was too risky to attempt to swim out to the jumper, so he came back to the bank and we tried to figure out what to do.

Someone on the truck thought quickly and lowered the hose from the truck to the water. He told the jumper to wrap the hose around himself several times and then attempt to swim to our bank. He assured the man the crew on the bridge would try to hold the hose taut to prevent the man from going (and staying) under the water.

Police and medics arrived in the middle of this master plan. Neither of their crews were any more prepared than we were because they expected us to have our kits, so they couldn't do anything but remain on standby. The jumper tried to do that awkward paddle he continued upstream to stay in place, but it proved more difficult while attempting to swim across the river. I instructed him to lie flat on his back. The crew on the bridge backed up the truck, which dragged the hose and the jumper closer to our bank. I was able to take the rope bag and lasso the jumper. I pulled him to the bank and he was rapidly treated for hypothermia protocol and a broken arm.

I couldn't leave well enough alone because I was wet and freezing and hungry because this asshat decided to do this in the middle of supper, so I asked what was so bad about his life that made him want to end it.

He told me he decided to kill himself after his pregnant girlfriend admitted the child wasn't his, but his brother's.

Since most of the guys on our truck have been through bad divorces and tons of crap like that, we told the guy it was a dumb thing to try to kill himself over and to be glad he knew the kid wasn't his before he had to make 18 years of child support payments. Maybe it wasn't the best thing to say to the poor guy, but I think it worked.

The last time I heard from the guy, he had just graduated from welding school and was seeing a woman he met while he was at the pool. Jumping off that bridge made him want to learn how to swim. Imagine that.

--K.F.

Tennessee

A Triage Story

This was a conversation I had with a patient in triage one night.

Me: So, it says you're here tonight because you have a headache?

Patient: Yeah.

Me: Okay, how long have you had this headache?

Patient: All day. I need something for it.

Me: Have you recently hit your head? Have you experienced any other symptoms with the pain?

Patient: No. My head just hurts. I need you to give me something for it so I can go home. I don't want to be here all night. Last week I had to be here for five hours and I missed the UFC fight.

Me: Why were you here last week?

Patient: My tooth hurt. They finally gave me Dilaudid. I need that for my head.

Me: Okay. So, do you smoke, drink alcohol, or use illegal drugs?

Patient: Yeah.

Me: To which part?

Patient: All of them.

Me: Okay. So, last time you were here it says you smoke about a pack a day, drink—.

Patient: It's all the same. Look, I just need something for my headache. It's really bad right now. You know, can I go smoke before we go back?

Me: We're almost done here, and no. I can't let you smoke on hospital property, especially when you're a patient.

Patient: But they let me last week.

Me: Well, this is this week.

Patient: (Mumbles 'c-word' under his breath)

Me: Okay, your previous-surgery list is filled out, but something seems to have happened to past illnesses. Let's go over these real fast and we'll take you back.

Patient: FINE.

Me: Have you had chickenpox, smallpox, measles—.

Patient: The only things I've ever had were chickenpox and Down Syndrome.

Me, caught off guard: W-what?

Patient: Chickenpox and—.

Me: Yes, I heard the part about chickenpox. But what was the other?

Patient: Down Syndrome.

Me: Down Syndrome?

Patient: Yeah. I had it when I was little. It was bad.

Me: And, uh, so what happened?

Patient: I don't know. My mom gave me Tylenol or something and it went away.

Every single time I think about this guy going around to all the different hospitals, trying to get drugs, and telling them he had Down Syndrome as a child, I crack up. I wonder if he goes around telling his girlfriends about that one time he was young and had it?

--P.H.

New York

I was prepping a woman for her first 8-week ultrasound and she asked me how long she had to wait to know what color the baby would be because she had cheated on her boyfriend and didn't know if it was his baby or her lover's.

My response was, "About seven more months."

--W.B.

Virginia

Please Be More Specific

Kerry, back in the day I worked in the ER as a unit clerk. We were also responsible for registering incoming patients, updating charts by hand (yes, it really was back in the day!), and communicating with our nurses incoming patients.

During one evening shift, a man walked inside. He was bundled up in an excessively large bubble overcoat. I didn't think much of it because it was cold here, following a rather serious blizzard that left us with about eleven feet of snow in two days. It was so bad that several of our doctors had not been home since the snow fell because they were unable to make the drives.

Anyway, I asked the man for his complaint and he told me his chest ached. He did not complain, nor did he act pained. I explained we were not only shorthanded, but due to the weather and influx of patients, we were also full. I'm not sure there was a single bed available in the entire hospital. The man was charmingly polite and said it was no problem at all, that he would take a seat in the waiting room and wait to be called. I watched him head to the waiting room, and he picked up a magazine. He flipped through a few of them from the coffee table over the course of an hour before a nurse came out and called for him.

I remember this nurse quite well because she was pregnant with twins and was as large as a house, ready to 'pop' any day. She was as sweet as could be and was a devote Catholic. Nothing ever seemed to get under her skin. She never had a bad word to say about anyone, no matter how much they did her wrong, and I'd never heard this sweet woman even begin to utter a cuss.

When the man with chest pain approached this nurse, he removed his jacket in preparation of his exam and that kind nurse yelled out the loudest four-letter-s-word I'd ever heard. I moved to cup my hand over the mouthpiece of the phone and turned my head to make sure she wasn't in labor, but then I saw what she had seen and I shouted for help.

What the man had neglected to tell me was his chest pain did not stem from a typical coronary complaint. He had a serrated meat knife jammed in his chest so deep that only the wooden handle was visible. This man sat in the waiting room with a knife protruding from his chest for an hour.

When he was rushed to the only open room in our ER, he told the doctors he had gotten in a fight with his brother, whom in return stabbed him. He requested that we did not call the police because his brother was on the force. We complied with his wishes.

The knife was six inches long and missed the patient's heart by a little more than one-half an inch. It was truly miraculous that the patient suffered no major damage or that the blade did not pierce an artery. He went to surgery and was admitted for a week, but then he was discharged with no complications.

I don't know what happened to this man when he left the hospital, but shortly after the pregnant nurse saw the knife she did give birth to her twins. We still think that the shock of the man's injury sent her in labor, and she's made a few jokes about the situation over the years. We always ribbed with her, telling her she should have named one of the boys Butcher or something along the lines of knives, but she and her husband decided to stick with their religious names.

--M.A.
Ohio

A woman once brought her dog to the ER at 3 AM because the vet was closed and she wanted 'solid answers' on why the dog was farting so much.

--K.K.

Connecticut

Real chief complaint from a 93-year-old SNF patient:

'I have no pulse and I think I'm dead.'

She refused to return to the SNF until we paged Cardio to confirm that she did, in fact, have a pulse and therefore was very much alive.

--P.B.

Hawaii

Dear parents,

No, I don't know if school was canceled or postponed. No, I can't call you if I hear anything. No, I can't tell you the weather forecast. No, I can't 'just talk' to your child and tell him/her to scare him/her into behaving 'this close to Christmas.' Because I am on the line telling you things that you, as an adult, should already know better than to ask of me, I am unable to help the driver trapped in his burning vehicle. Please stop calling 911 with stupid questions when you could go on Facebook or listen to the radio for answers.

--O.E.
Idaho

Lowest of the Low

This is a story about hospital drama, not a story about a patient.

I worked as a registrar and on any given shift, there were probably two to three other women on duty besides myself. We mostly got along, but then a new girl was hired.

First off, this girl lied about being pregnant so she could get the job. I understand rationality behind that, and I understand that pregnancy is not a disability, but maybe someone should have told the girl this because she would work for a few minutes (yes, minutes) and then believe she was entitled to take the rest of the shift to sit at our desk and text her husband.

We all grumbled throughout her pregnancy, through all of her short-or-no-notice call-ins, through what work she was doing being done incorrectly. Of course, you could tell management all of these things all day long, but they really didn't care. They said it was part of 'teamwork,' to carry each other. The way I saw it, the rest of us weren't getting a cut of the girl's pay to be a 'team,' but whatever.

Anyway, the girl took off two months early for maternity leave because she found a loophole in the HR maternity policy. Then she was gone her traditional eight weeks of our hospital's maternity leave. During this time, she came in frequently to be seen for the dumbest stuff, herself becoming a frequent flyer. It's pretty bad when you work there and people know you're a frequent. She always requested one male doctor, a man probably three times her age who was happily married for decades and had grown children, grandchildren, and great-grandchildren. He was an all-around nice, moral man and I've never seen him treat anyone poorly, even if they deserved it. The girl would become upset if she couldn't get the doctor she requested, sometimes to the point of crying so hard she made herself throw up, or other times she'd become so angry that she threatened nurses. It was embarrassing for all of us. When the ER nurses started complaining to

HR about the girl's behavior, they said they couldn't terminate someone on maternity leave and blamed the girl's hormones for her behavior. Again, she was pretty much allowed to do what she wanted, and the rest of us were fed up.

The girl was scheduled to come back after four months of half-paid/half-unpaid maternity leave, but-SURPRISE!-she found another loophole in the system and got to take another four weeks off as short-term disability, where she was paid for more time off. She would come in as a patient, bragging about how she knew when she first started the job that she would be able to do this, and it was one of the reasons she applied at the hospital. She bragged about doing the same thing during her two other pregnancies at different employers. This made a lot of us frustrated because you don't want to hear someone boasting about not working and still getting paid when you have someone's puke on your shirt.

When the girl *finally* came back to work, she settled right back in as the lazy coworker. Now, though, she was obsessed with that doctor she kept coming in to see after she had the baby.

One night, we were not busy and the girl was asking us all how to go about stealing a married man from his wife. One of the techs heard this and explained you can't *really* steal a man, that he has to go willingly, and that if a man is happy with his current partner, it's unlikely that he's going to be going anywhere. The girl didn't like that answer, so she accused the tech of sexually harassing her. It was her word against his, but he was fired to avoid liability. It made everyone livid, especially because the tech was gay, with zero interest in women sexually. Seriously, the guy saw a picture of a vagina one time and he puked in the trash can.

After this, the girl began dressing differently for work. While the rest of us would be in business slacks and nice blouses, she would come in decked out in a dress with heels and full make up like she was about to go to someone's wedding. She went to the ER room area to 'work,' but work would pile up on us and we'd catch her sitting next to the doctor she was crushing on, just chatting away. On his end, it appeared casual. On her end, you could see the little heart-shaped-flames in her eyes.

Well, one night, the girl told us she had a plan to get the doctor to 'fall for' her. She called her husband and said she didn't need a ride home because one of us said we'd take her. Then she worked up some fake tears, went to the doctor, and told him she didn't have a ride home. He gave her a ride.

All the next day, we had to listen to the girl telling us how she and the doctor just chatted away during the entire ride home and how she thought he was interested in her and blah, blah, blah. She even had a little nickname for him now. It was sickening. But when the doctor walked in for a call-in, he didn't even make eye contact with the girl or say anything. Of course, this made her mad.

The girl continued flirting with the doctor and he routinely gave her rides home for almost a week. Then it was time for the girl to make her move. We found her searching online for seductive sexual advances and she showed us all how she had divorce papers drawn up because she was now set on having this doctor's baby and 'having it made.'

We went to management with this, but it was brushed under the rug. I don't know how a tech could get accused of sexual harassment, but this girl could do everything she did and still be hired, but that was the case. Nobody knew whether to say anything to the doctors, and by this point, even the nurses knew what the girl was up to. At the front desk, we decided that the doctor was a grown man and if he wanted to cheat on his wife, there really wasn't anything we could do.

On the night the girl went around telling all of us that she wasn't wearing panties and packed flavored lubricant in her bag so she could perform oral on the doctor as he was driving her home, she went back with her tears to ask him for a ride. I was talking to another nurse at the time and saw the whole thing unfold.

First, the girl leaned over the counter to start her conversation with the doctor. Then, he gave her a tissue and told her life was too short for tears. I rolled my eyes.

Well, the girl sat next to the doctor like she'd done so many times before and went on to ask for her ride. He agreed to give her a ride home and the talk went from that to small-talk, which was her flirting heavily and him telling corny jokes about farm animals, the kind of jokes you'd tell to your small children. (What do you call a cow whose baby ran away? De-calf-einated.)

The girl cackled at the doctor's jokes and then she touched his arm and said, "Oh, I just love your jokes. You are just too funny, sweetheart."

Half of the nurses were eyeing in their direction, just in time to see the doctor's face grow red as a beet. He jerked his arm away from the girl and said, "My name is not *sweetheart.* It is *Doctor* X, and that is the *only* way you will address me in this emergency room or anyplace else."

He went on to blast her in front of everyone, saying he was happily married and had been doing her a favor by giving her a ride home because he knew she was young and had children. We had no reason to believe the doctor was being insincere with his words. He told the girl he wouldn't go to HR with a complaint, but she needed to get over her 'fantasy' and remain at a distance from him, only to communicate with him professionally.

The next day, the girl was late to work, but not her 'typical' lateness. This time she was two hours late, meaning I had to come in early and another person had to stay over until we could figure something out. When the girl came in, she sat around and did nothing. Finally, after an hour of this, she just randomly decided to pick up the phone, call our boss, and tell our boss she was quitting because she was tired of being the only one in our department doing any work. Then she walked out in the middle of her shift.

The rest of us were called to a mandatory departmental meeting, where we were lectured and scolded on 'teamwork' and how it was our fault that we lost an employee and now we were going to have to 'wait it out' until we could find a replacement for the girl. That meeting made a lot of people mad and two of us put in our notices of resignation at the end of the meeting.

I work as a secretary now, and I can tell you I definitely don't miss all the drama that happened around the ER.

Oh, I still see that girl around town. She received a settlement from a bank after she said she was sexually harassed, and now she's pregnant again (and on paid leave).

Some things never change.

-P.F.

Indiana

A man brought his son in this one time and the only thing he could tell us was, "My wife told me to bring him here." The kid didn't have a fever, had no pain complaints, and dad didn't know if there were any recent falls or head bumps.

We told the man to call his wife to find out why she thought her kid needed to be in the ER at midnight, but he couldn't reach her so he just went back home.

--T.N.

Minnesota

Taking Time to Talk

I am contracted with a suburban hospital with roughly 500 beds within the entire facility, excluding beds found on the mental health ward. We see hundreds of patients in the ED each day, yet our patients come in and expect us to recall every conversation we have ever had, every visit off the top of our heads, and often become frustrated when we can't treat them like Joe the Butcher welcoming back his best lamb consumer.

Once such case of this occurring was a 63-year-old woman brought in via EMS for a probable GI bleed. She complained of melena (dark stools) and hematemesis (blood detected in vomiting/vomiting blood). She additionally complained of midline abdominal discomfort.

Right off the bat, this woman was frustrated with me because I did not know her name without looking at her chart. She was foul-mouthed and I tried to ignore her crassness because it had been a long day already.

I largely ignored the woman's conversation unless it pertained to her medical history and explained I was doing so due to her poor attitude and behavior. Upon this point, the patient hurled a bed pan in my direction; it hit my scribe in the head and she needed sutures for the wound.

This patient found my lack of remembrance to be rude and she refused to allow me to examine her. I informed the patient that she was more than welcome to request another physician, and that there are times staff and patients simply do not interact well enough to offer the patient the workup he or she deserves and/or desires. This frustrated my patient even further, and it was futile to even attempt to reason with her or enter her room again. She actively refused to answer any questions or allow myself or my RNs to examine her. Essentially, she was a sitting duck in a rather-busy ER.

To open the lines of communication with this patient, my staff had to pull up all the patient's past records. I learned I treated this same patient two years prior. The patient was not remotely interested in hearing that we knew her medical history, but as soon as personal notes charted by the RNs in the past were read back to the patient, she opened up and said, "See, I knew you remembered me."

We continued detailing the patient's symptoms. The key to any proper diagnosis is to interact with your patients on their level. This patient did not wish to discuss her medical history or symptoms medically, so I related to her on a personal level and asked about her day-to-day life. In the forty-five minutes it took to listen to her recall her week at bingo, visiting her grandchildren, and finding a gentleman to fix her flat tire, I also learned the patient had been consuming a rather large quantity of bismuth subsalicylate (Pepto Bismol) to self-treat daily heartburn. Another noteworthy portion of her story was how dry she said the air in her home was.

Through a conversation regarding the patient's personal life, I learned this woman was not suffering from a GI bleed. The dry air in her living environment irritated her sinuses, and the large consumption of bismuth subsalicylate irritated her stomach lining and darkened her stools. When she vomited, her sinuses would bleed, mimicking hematemesis.

On a hunch, I wanted to further examine the patient's complaint of daily heartburn. Following extensive testing, the patient was diagnosed with heart disease.

I plead of all patients, physicians included, not to self-medicate. Any attempt to do so may interact with an underlying cause and, like this patient, make your true diagnosis one to miss. I owe the patient's attitude thankfulness because without it I would not have been frustrated enough to approach her on a different level, meaning I would have misdiagnosed her.

--J.W., M.D.
North Carolina

Pass the Sauce

This is the only story I received by multiple staff. These RNs, registration clerks, and surg techs share my books within their circles, and I greatly appreciate that! Now, on to the, uh, *remarkable* story.

It was about two in the morning when this guy walked in. And when I say he walked in, he really walked. He wasn't moving funny. He wasn't breathing weird. He just walked.

I asked him if he needed to be seen in the ER and he made some wisecrack about if he didn't need to be seen he wouldn't be there, so I asked him for his name and information. He was a new patient, so I filled out all his information and made copies of his insurance card.

When I asked him for a chief complaint, his face turned red and he laughed awkwardly, like he just told a dirty joke to himself but it was a nasty one so he didn't know how to react.

Like you said in your books a thousand times, I've heard it all. I've been in this job for four years now, and I feel like there's nothing I haven't seen or heard or been called by angry patients. I told the man there was nothing to be embarrassed about and no matter how bad he thought it was, the nurses have dealt with everything.

Then the man told me he had a bottle stuck in his rectum.

I had to send the man to the waiting room while I went to find the triage nurse. I didn't ask what kind of bottle it was.

(Second submission:) Triage walked my patient to a room to allow him to lie down. I'm sure you've seen this occur several times. It is not uncommon here, either. I waited until the triage nurse completed her questioning and she approached me for a report. She could not keep a straight face, so I started feeling irritated because I was having a horrible night and was exhausted.

When I asked triage what was so funny, she told me the patient complained of a soy sauce bottle in his rectum. He and his partner had been experimenting, but the body's natural suction (it's a real thing) grasped the glass and the patient could not remove the bottle from his anus.

Two doctors and I attempted to remove the bottle using forceps, but it was really lodged deep and firm. The patient's crying did not make this any easier. He repeatedly stated that his ex-wife worked upstairs and if she found out he would never hear the end of it. He did not seem concerned about what anybody else thought. He apologized many times throughout the extraction attempt. He cried harder when I told him the bad news: he had to go to surgery.

(Third submission;) My job is to stand in the corner and look pretty. Just kidding. I am basically the person the surgeon yells at if he has to turn his head to look for a piece of equipment. I also get yelled at if we're having a surgery and the doctor requires equipment that we would not use on that surgery and it's not automatically there. Basically, it's like if you give someone soup for an appetizer and they yell at you because you didn't serve the soup with a steak knife. That's my job, to anticipate that the surgeon's tray needs a steak knife to serve with his soup.

The guy we received from the ER was sedated on the cot when I walked by the operating room. Two surgeons were present. One was there as a standby. I was present to hand off equipment to the surgeon. He had two nurses. The anesthesia tech was there.

I'll spare all the details, but let me say that putting the guy under was the easy part. I think I'm in the wrong field because I'd love to tell a guy to count backwards from ten and he passes out at six and then I just made a thousand dollars.

When the surgeon opened this guy up, there was a Kikkoman soy sauce bottle (low sodium) stuck in this guy. The surgeon tried to remove it by irrigating its surroundings and giving it a light tug. When he did, the cap came off the bottle. There was soy sauce spilling all over the patient's insides.

We thought the surgery was going to take maybe an hour, hour-and-a-half, tops. Because we had to spend at least that irrigating soy sauce and trying to remove the cap from the man's organs, the surgery lasted about three hours.

The only good news I have, you know, other than the surgeon removing the bottle from the patient, is that I didn't get yelled at once because the surgeon was too busy laughing.

(Fourth submission:) CCU received a patient from surgery. Everyone on the floor knew why he was a patient and thought it was hilarious, but we remained professional to the patient's face and giggled about it at our desks. The patient was not overly needy. He kept asking if he had visitors.

When I returned to work that night, the patient was still in recovery. His partner was in the room with him. They were loudly arguing over which one of them thought sticking the bottle up his rear end was a good idea. We had to call security because they wouldn't stop yelling at each other.

The patient was discharged the next day, with orders to remain on light duty only and to refrain from sexual participation for at least six weeks. He and his partner argued over that, too.

--All names and location withheld at submitters' requests.

<u>End of Watch</u>

Kerry, I enjoy your books and need to ask if you can do me a favor. Please tell my story. It might help others grieving or save a life.

My husband and I met in high school, and we had that stereotypical 'young love' thing going on. We had difficulty conceiving, but we promised we'd never stop trying. My husband felt a calling for the police force and went for it. He was away for training camp for six weeks, and as he dedicated himself to the job, he would miss family dinners, holidays, have to leave in the middle of a movie if he was called away, and he did not get a lot of sleep if something particularly bad happened. Still, he was the best husband anyone could ask for.

He was the first responder at a frozen lake many years ago. He was always the kind of person who would gladly give you the shirt off his back if that meant you would stay a little warmer and more comfortable. That's just the kind of person he was. So, when he heard from a group of children that two of their friends had fallen through the ice, he didn't wait. He rushed out on the ice and could reach the first child. She was conscious and breathing, so he moved her to the bank and gave her his jacket until paramedics arrived on scene.

While the first child was safe, the second was not. My husband could not see the second child in the water where the ice had broken. He eventually spotted the child's red coat against the ice a few feet down and ran down that direction, but he couldn't break the ice. He tried so hard that he broke his hand in the process. He was finally able to break a chunk free and grab the child, but it was too late. He held the boy's head above water until help arrived to remove the child's body from the water, afraid that if he let go the child's body would be swept away or be pulled to the bottom of the lake.

This incident left my husband devastated. He became a shell of his former self. He withdrew from life. He no longer found interest in hobbies. He removed himself from on-call volunteer lists at work. One time, when we heard a call over the radio, he shook his head and said, "It's not like it'll make a difference if we're there or not."

My husband refused counseling because we're from a rural area and he said it just 'wasn't what the guys would do.' Everyone acted like nothing happened when they'd come around.

Seven months following the accident at the lake, my husband shot himself. We had been married thirteen wonderful years. I walked through the front door expecting an answer when I asked what he wanted for dinner, and then my world ended when I walked in our bedroom. He left a note that begged everyone in his life to forgive him. It said he felt worthless that he could not save the child at the lake, and if he couldn't save that child, he couldn't save himself.

I've been without my husband for fifteen years and miss him each day. I refuse to remarry.

From my husband's death, I learned there is a suicide in our emergency responder family each day, but I don't pay mind to statistics because my husband was not a number and neither are any of his veterans from the department. I have forgiven myself for not doing more or seeing his emotional breakdown for what it really was, but if I could go back with what I know now, I would have tried to help, tried to recognize the beginning stages of depression.

PTSD and thoughts of suicide, I've learned, are high in the first responders field, and how can it not be? How can we expect anyone to lift a charred body from an extinguished vehicle to a body bag for transport to the morgue without that haunting them? How can we expect our husbands, wives, and friends to forget the face of the man shot in front of him?

It's true that not everyone is cut out for the police department, paramedics, fire department, or hospital setting. I worked in the ER for the first three years of my marriage and would never want to go back to something like that because I'm not cut for that line of work and seeing what they see there. It's not unreasonable to stop asking our law enforcement and emergency responders to carry such heavy loads. There is a stigma related to these professions, one that says it's not okay to talk about emotions or how the scene affected them, that they should hold it all in and let it kill them from the inside out. We must end that stigma and let our police and emergency responders' families know that it's okay to breakdown, and it's okay to talk about feelings.

--L.R.

Wyoming

A Message to Readers

Oh people, you're killing me with these submissions! They're wild, they're shocking, they're sad, they're miraculous.

First off, I would like to again thank all my readers, new or dedicated. I am grateful to have such an amazing audience, and I do enjoy hearing from you guys in reviews, on Twitter, or on Facebook (though it still takes me a while to meander on over that direction). You are all polite and supportive, and I am blessed to have you in my corner.

Secondly, I want to add that none of these submissions were paid. It was explained and agreed upon that stories used would not be compensated. There was no incentive or favoritism or any bribery involved with this compilation of stories, just simply readers wishing to share experiences.

Now, I am currently out of the hospital scene. If it's temporary or permanent, who knows. As far as my writing career is concerned, I thought long and hard about piecing together this book. I am actively working on other pieces of (non-hospital) fiction. Everything's a work in progress, though, so again, who knows. I'm trying to thoroughly enjoy my life and take one thing at a time.

Several readers have mentioned in reviews that they were unable to load my books. Please note that this does not appear to be an error on this end. I've been unable to determine a fix for this. If you purchased a copy you cannot read, please submit a ticket to the place that sold you the copy. You shouldn't have to pay for something you can't read.

As usual, if you notice errors, have questions, just want to comment…I read all reviews and am active on Twitter. You can also 'like' my page 'Author Kerry Hamm' on Facebook, but I still am slow to jump over there, so response times won't be nearly as fast.

Please continue to be your fabulous selves and one last time, THANK YOU for reading!

I appreciate you more than you will ever know.

Merry Christmas and Happy New Year!

Check me out on Twitter!

https://twitter.com/AuthorKerryHamm

www.ingramcontent.com/pod-product-compliance
Lightning Source LLC
Chambersburg PA
CBHW071416180526
45170CB00001B/117